THE RESISTED EXERCISE

THE RESISTED EXERCISE

A PHYSIO'S STORY

by

AUDREY B. INSLEY

The Memoir Club

First published in 2012 by
The Memoir Club
Arya House
Langley Park
Durham
DH7 9XE
Tel: 0191 373 5660
Email: memoirclub@msn.com

British Library Cataloguing in
Publication Data.
A catalogue record for this book
is available from the
British Library

ISBN: 978-1-84104-543-6

Printed by HPM Group, Newton Aycliffe, Co Durham

For my Sons: Rowan and Haydn
&
Grandchildren: Elizabeth and William

With my love as and for always

And, of course, for H.

'Brilliant Grandpa'

Contents

Acknowledgement

I would like to express my gratitude to my editor,
John Shaw, for his unfailing help and support while writing this book.

Foreword

When I was asked to write the foreword to this book, I was made aware of the journey that the profession of Physiotherapy itself has taken in that time.

It is nearly sixty years since those student days Then nearly all training took place in the general hospital with additional lectures at the Manchester School of Medicine. As students they were let loose on the unsuspecting public after a mere three months as assistants to the qualified staff in the well-known adage that nothing teaches as well as practice. Based at a busy city hospital, they were sent to various specialist hospitals to widen their experience, giving them a glimpse of the many specialities into which they might enter on qualification.

As science is not static, many advances have been made in diagnostic tools enabling far more effective treatment. The increase in biometrics has produced more efficient use of the human body, particularly in the area of sport, which guards against injury and maximises ability.

In both the Olympics and Para-Olympics, teams of physiotherapists were permanently on duty, aiding the athletes to stay in peak condition hopefully through to the finals and medals. In the equestrian events, the physiotherapists treated both human and equestrian athletes.

The many boundaries of medicine have been extended by all members of the medical world particularly, in war arenas. Physiotherapists have been required to be ground breaking in their treatments to enable both service personnel and civilians to return as active, valued members of the community as soon as possible.

Finally, this book tells the story of young people, their careers and lives within the hospital community and outside it. It is hoped that many such people, interested in a life of service to others, will continue to take up the many and varied opportunities offered worldwide, by the profession of Physiotherapy.

T.C

CHAPTER ONE

Sacked

We were on a bus sitting side by side – not speaking. It was soon after eight, on a bright, chilly morning. My father and I were travelling into the centre of Manchester, towards my father's place of business in the ancient quarter of the city known as Hanging Ditch, while I was to start life as a physiotherapy student, for the second time.

Exactly a year before, I had set out to join fellow first year students in the physiotherapy school in the city of Salford, next door to Manchester. I had been there five or six weeks when, out of the blue, the Principal sent for me. I approached her office with some trepidation, she was that sort of person and I had no idea why I had been summoned to the holy of holies. I knocked on the door, straining my ears for the 'come in'. As soon as I heard the voice I turned the door handle and entered.

'Come in Miss Arden' she said. 'I have just heard from London regarding your entrance qualifications, they can find no trace of physics and neither can I.'

'No that's correct,' I responded 'I did explain to you at the time.'

'Yes, I'm sure you did, but London say it is imperative and I'm afraid it is out of my hands and you cannot continue until you get that A level, I am most awfully sorry but you will have to leave.'

And that was that! I was completely stunned. How could that have happened? I thought as I opened the door and let myself out. I had entered the office a physiotherapy student and left as a dazed nobody.

I went to collect my things and left the hospital as quickly as possible. I had no wish to meet anybody at all.

My parents listened to my story with growing dismay and consternation. They contacted the school and did everything possible to get the decision reversed, all to no avail. So there I was, in the middle of November out on the academic street. I had a straight choice of either cramming for the exam next May or forgetting once and for all that I wanted to become a physiotherapist.

Not surprisingly, I wanted to forget the whole nightmare.

I spent a very tearful next few days trying to decide just what to do. I had always wanted to do physiotherapy and now what to do instead? I was like a rudderless ship.

After a seemingly hopeless and weepy week, my father decided something had to be done. He told me he had spoken to my cousin at the Town Hall in Manchester, where she was in charge of catering and had explained the situation to her and she had offered me a part time job. I knew she had only offered it to me to please my father, of whom she was very fond. She certainly didn't have much time for me and normally would not have entertained the idea of a relative working for her anyway.

'The plan is' continued my father, 'for you to cram for your exam in the morning and to work for Norah from noon until four in the afternoon. When you know your exam results in the summer, then, you can make your decision.'

As I expected, working for Norah proved to be no picnic either. She was rightly adamant that no favouritism should be shown to me, and it wasn't.

The kitchen supervisor was suspicious of me from the start, she kept me busy and within her sight the whole time. I was given the 'central station,' in the kitchen, to keep clean. It was a nightmare. It was the area under and around the giant chip pans. Everything to be deep fried was based there. At one time the floor surface had been smooth and fairly easy to clean but with repeated scrubbing the surface had become porous and pitted. The holes in the surface filled with grease from the deep pans and the only method of removing it was to pour boiling water over the surface, melting the fat then wiping away the greasy liquid before it congealed again. Only now could I clean the floor. Before the first week was out I had two rows of massive blisters across each palm of my very swollen hands.

Another part of my job, the supervisor informed me, was to collect and carry all the dirty pans, cooking trays and containers and deliver them to the 'washer-up.' Mrs Haslam was the veritable Trojan, whose sole job it was to scour and clean these huge vessels. Rebecca Haslam or Bekky, as she was known to everyone, was sixty if she was a day and probably nearer seventy. My girls never retire, they are far too loyal my cousin had told me, and it did seem to be the case with one or two of her 'girls.' Bekky was short, about four foot ten inches (147cm) and dumpy in build. She had lost all her teeth except for two and both were yellow. Her thin and grey wispy hair was scraped back into a knot at the back of her head. To do her work, she stood on a specially built wooden duckboard so she could reach into the great troughs of hot water, one for washing the other for rinsing. The mountains of dirty receptacles would be stacked and piled high on her right hand side until there didn't seem room for anything else.

I would come along with my arms full and stack them even higher. On my first day I had serious misgivings about the safety of these mountains, Bekky seemed in danger from avalanches of old gravy and custard. Where should I put this load I had asked her anxiously? Bekky, turned to me, took her reddened hands out of the water and carefully wiped them down her apron of sacking which she wore to 'save' her overall.

'If tha can't find a place tha'd better stand and ole em,' she said and fiercely wrenched off a huge piece of wire wool from a great role, setting my teeth on edge.

Bekky never spoke much and, when I got to know her better, I realised she had made quite a speech to me on my first day. Every day I would bring load upon load, she wouldn't say anything, just nod as the next delivery was made. One morning though I did hear Bekky speak and pretty forthrightly too. It was to a waitress who brought a tray of huge carving knives to 'Bekky's station,' seeing the huge stack of dirty pans waiting to be washed she emptied the tray straight into the sudsy water. Bekky who was sitting a few paces away, sucking appreciatively at a well-earned cup of tea watched this fool.

'Cum back 'ere' Bekky roared – the whole kitchen froze. Everyone stopped and watched including the hapless waitress who had no idea she was at fault. 'You dropped all them cleavers in there! So you can put your 'ands in and get 'em out again, I'm not getting cut ta pieces for you or anyone else!' With that she resumed supping her tea, all the while her beady eyes on the silly woman groping about gingerly, up to her elbows in deep soapy water trying to fish out the sabre sharp knives. Nobody ever did that to Bekky again.

All day, every day, Bekky would clean and scour, moving the used mountain of dirty pans from her right hand side through one sink to another finally ending up with a gleaming mountain of pans on her left hand side. She worked steadily with the dedication of a saint and everyone respected her.

Meanwhile, each morning, I was attending a tutorial college in the city; no more than a five minute brisk walk to work. I was supposed to attend nine until twelve noon but I left a little early to be at the Town Hall promptly.

The tutor was a young fellow, not long after graduation himself and there were about twelve of us in the class. The sessions were pleasant enough but there was certainly no sense of exam urgency about them and as they were costing my parents ill-afforded fees, I knew it was up to me to study hard at night. It was tiring but at least there was a plan, I was no longer in a state of flux and I could not let my parents down.

A few days after starting work at the Town Hall, we were having dinner at home when my mother suddenly asked me to show her my hands. I put down my knife and fork and turned my palms upwards. The two rows of huge blisters on each hand, which had developed in the first couple of days, were now replaced by two rows of sturdy segs. The double rows of callous were not a pretty sight and I quickly picked up my knife and fork and started eating again but not before my mother had looked at my father who was gazing at my hands in silent horror.

Next day I arrived at work to find a very angry cousin on the warpath. She was waiting for me the centre of the kitchen, where a lot of eyes were watching, and she said accusingly, 'I have just had your father on the phone, show me your hands!' I stood there, like a five-year-old, while she examined my hands. 'Why didn't you speak to me yourself?' She asked crossly, clearly thinking I was a tell-tale. It was no use trying to explain, she was in a tearing hurry as usual. And before I could think of anything in my defence, she was off calling over her shoulder 'I'll find something else for you tomorrow.' I hurried away to start work mortified by the several onlookers watching for my reaction.

Next day I was elevated to the heady height of being a waitress in the separate councillors' dining room. I was to be responsible for running this special room and there would be a young waitress to help me, 'so get on with it' my cousin said briskly.

The councillors' dining room had a quiet, confidential air, where private council matters were discretely discussed, the conversation muffled by the thick grey carpet and heavy maroon curtains. The two beautiful mahogany dining tables were surrounded by handsome chairs, their maroon leather, beautifully tooled in gold with the city crest. There was one larger table set apart from the others, curtained off in an alcove. This private space was for the Town clerk and the five or six or so senior heads of departments such as the Head of Transport, the Head of Parks or Head of Utilities and other city fathers.

Philip Dingle was the Town Clerk in those days, and judging by the frequency he chose it, grilled plaice was his favourite meal. He was also incredibly fond of tomato sauce which he applied so liberally whatever meal he had ordered looked more like something out of 'Custer's last stand,' rather than a dish that had been specially prepared for him.

Working as a waitress, my pay was reduced because, as we were told, 'your pay will be augmented by your tips.' Gladys, my helper, and I soon found tipping was directly related to politics in the Councillors' dining room. The further left wing the councillor was, the less they tipped until the 'extreme left,' never tipped at all. Obviously those pundits who had worked out our pay scales had never worked in a Councillors dining room. At the end of the day, Gladys and I would count up our tips such as they were. They meant a great deal to both of us, I, to save for when I was a student again, if ever, and Gladys, who was newly engaged was busy saving up to get married.

I got on well with Gladys. After every one had gone and we had tidied the place up, we would sit down and enjoy a cup of tea together. I would listen as she told me of her wedding plans. It was to be just a quiet wedding but it has to be in church she had said earnestly.

Gladys was a pleasant person, quite happy with her lot in life and particularly with her Alfred. Together they were both saving up in both furniture and clothing 'clubs' ready for when they were given the keys to their council flat. Gladys was only two years older than me but in many ways she was my elder by light years. I would listen attentively as she talked of the mysteries of going to the housing department 'to put our name down,' or how her Alfred always treated her to a rum and pep whenever she was off colour, down at 'The Crown.' I had been raised a Quaker and had never been in a pub in my life. When I eventually left the Town hall, I missed Gladys and her everyday tales of city life.

CHAPTER TWO

Reluctant Return

It was the beginning of October, term was starting, and in the summer, I had managed to get the relevant qualification required by The Chartered Society of Physiotherapy.

The bus pulled into the terminus and we rose to get off. My father sensing my mood and the reluctance I was feeling said, 'just give it a try, if you don't like it you don't have to continue.' With that he kissed me goodbye and walked off to his place of work.

Those few words made all the difference to me. Our family were not well-off and because I had chosen the three-and-a-half-year course in physiotherapy, my grant was very small, just enough to pay my fees and books. It did not pay for my uniform or anything else. It left me with just five shillings a week (25 pence) for bus fares and anything else I required. I felt heavily burdened. So when my father had said that I should give it six months and if I didn't want to continue not to worry, a great load seemed to be lifted from my shoulders. But that did not mean I was looking forward to returning, I was not. My original colleagues would now be a year ahead and they no doubt would be feeling their superiority.

I crossed the road and stepped into Marks and Spencer's. As it was our first day we were not due at the hospital until ten, that just gave me time to buy some necessities.

I needed some navy pants. During training, physio students spend a great deal of time in their underwear being practised upon and it was advisable if not mandatory, to have practical rather than alluring knickers. It was a measure of my reluctance to return to the fold that I had left the purchase of such items until the last minute. Having made my purchase I hurried off to Salford, a City that adjoins Manchester just across the river Irwell. The hospital was a good fifteen minutes, brisk walk away, I had to hurry, no money to waste on bus fares.

I headed off and joined Chapel Street, the main London to Carlisle A6 road. There as usual, was the tall policeman, on point duty, looking even taller in his helmet. The road was hugely busy with traffic joining this intersection from all directions especially to and from Manchester, yet this stately, unruffled, greatly skilled officer always kept the dense traffic moving smoothly by his seemingly, unhurried movements.

I passed the Roman Catholic Cathedral and there next door, was Salford Royal Hospital where I was to be based. To the side of the hospital steps there was an ugly, new square brick building. On the wall, to the side of the front door was a plaque dedicated to the memory of the fourteen girls who had been killed in a bombing raid, during the Second World War, on their very first day in nursing school. The far side of the hospital looked over the grand curve of the river Irwell with the crescent of its lovely Georgian houses.

No time for that now I told myself and dashed up the front steps, down the corridor, across the quad and into the medical gym where the introductory lecture was being held. I pushed open the door there was a moments silence as 'Bo' the head of school cut off mid-sentence, all eyes were on me. I was late she said so, hardly an auspicious second start.

I meekly sat down and listened to the familiar talk on the proposed timetable and the fact that both male and female students would share all lectures including practical sessions with the strict exception of those of manipulation and massage!

My eyes went round the familiar medical gym. It was smaller than the huge general one at Salford Lads Club, which we went to down the road at the back of the hospital. The medical gym was used to give patients individual treatments or to give classes to small groups of patients with the same medical conditions. It was furnished with plinths, slings and pulleys, walking aids, static bicycles and portable flights of stairs, mats and all the rest of impedimenta required for a rehab unit. It also contained desks so it doubled as a lecture theatre. Space was at a premium in this old hospital.

In the corner of this room, stood a literature stand, still displaying, though seemingly never read, all manner of booklets published by the Catholic Truth Society. Bo or Miss Bodoano, as she was more correctly known, was a keen Roman Catholic. It was not coincidental that most of the female students were Roman Catholics - coming from the safe haven of six form convents. Needless to say that I, a Quaker, was pretty much beyond the pale and certainly of doubtful religious origins as far as Bo was concerned. It was all very non-politically correct in those days. One poor student on introducing herself to Bo confessed to her that although she had been born a catholic she had later been received into the Church of England. Bo had stood there, mouth pursed, eyebrows twitching, the silence palpable. She didn't last long.

The majority of the male students were older than most of us, having done their two years National Service. There were some Manchester United footballers, doing the three year course in six years so that they could study in the then non football season. Footballers were not as well paid as they are today and these male students were trying to secure their future in what was often a short precarious profession. There were sacked medical students though why they had left was any bodies guess and rumours were rife. There was one guy, so legend had it, who had a traumatic love affair, went on a bender for a month and ended up a lighthouse keeper in some far flung Scottish corner. Eventually, sufficiently purged, he enrolled as a physio student at Salford.

While the lecture continued, I watched Bo. She had not changed in the last few months unsurprisingly. Her full name was Maria Theresa Bodoano, and it was fairly safely reputed that she was of Italian origin. Whether she was or not, she certainly looked as if she might have had Italian parents. Her eyes were black brown in colour and she had a dark rosy complexion. Bo was about five foot seven with a substantial torso that gave no hint of a waist. Her thin legs were somewhat angular, ending with long slender feet, which were always firmly planted at ten to two.

Bo had keen eyesight and had an unnerving habit of silently standing and watching , hands tucked firmly into her starched white belt, feet planted firmly apart, mouth twitching. I was later to find out, to my cost, this gimlet stare and mouth twitching was directly proportional to the hash you were making of things as you practised a treatment, mercifully, on a fellow student. Finally when she could not stand the incompetence, usually mine, any longer she would march over with a brisk 'stand aside.'

At last the introductory lecture was drawing to a close with Bo announcing our timetable for the first term. Along with anatomy and physiology, there were electro mechanics, pathology, physics and psychology. We would do medical gym to get future patients fit and regular gym to get us fit.

'You will do two weeks nursing as soon as it can be arranged,' Bo announced as an afterthought. 'So you will get used to treating inpatients.'

But would we live that long?

CHAPTER THREE

New Friends, New Language

We became proper students with the start of anatomy lectures. They took precedence over everything because as Miss Bently pointed out, 'you cannot treat patients unless you know what is deep to the skin.' She added as an afterthought, 'once you have learnt that, you have the tools of your profession for life.'

Ann Bently was a good looking woman in her late thirties with curly light brown hair that was going fetchingly grey. She had a lovely complexion that was heightened by her condition. It was rumoured Miss Bently had malignant hypertension and because of that she had turned down several offers of Headship. She certainly never appeared to hurry in her walking pace, which was deliberately slow nor did she ever raise her voice from the quiet tone, which she always used.

Ann Bently's knowledge of anatomy was formidable. She was a walking 'Gray's Anatomy,' that mighty tome that has informed medical students since it was first written by Henry Gray, a surgeon at St George's hospital in 1858 and which is even today, updated regularly by leading anatomists.

Miss Bently had a hidden talent for anatomy, which we were all blithely unaware of on our first day, all that is, except me who had been alerted to it last year. So when this gently spoken lecturer first appeared, she was met with a relaxed audience as she entered the lecture theatre. With one fluid movement she picked up a right scapula, took hold of the articulated skeleton with her left hand and began to speak with the rapidity of a machine gun. Everyone was taken off balance. There was a hasty scramble for writing implements as she spoke quickly, quietly and as we were to find out, always accurately. 'The scapula is a flat triangular bone lying on the posterolateral aspect of the chest wall, covering parts of the second to the seventh ribs. It presents for examination, costal, dorsal surfaces, upper, lateral and medial borders, superior, inferior, lateral angles and three bony, processes.' Miss Bently seemed to caress the bone as she pointed out the groove for the circumflex scapula artery before replacing the bone in its wooden box.

Our lecturer, looked solemnly round the room and said, 'you must be able to draw and describe the scapula and it relationships by tomorrow, good morning ladies and gentlemen.' With that she glided out, leaving a group of bemused innocents staring at the door.

Everyone continued to sit there in dazed silence; obviously before we could proceed we would have to learn a whole new vocabulary. 'And,' added the girl sitting next to me, 'it will have to be PDQ,' I looked enquiringly at my neighbour 'pretty damn quick' she said and I nodded in complete agreement.

This pleasant girl, was to become my great friend, her name was Fiona Gilway. She was attractive, curvy, five foot two in height with dark brown eyes. Her hair was equally dark and slightly wavy, it was secured up and out of the way by a discrete navy ribbon so the hair fell into a gentle corkscrewing 'pony tail.'

Fiona was Roman Catholic and brought up in the strict confines of a convent boarding school from which she had emerged with a heightened sense of humour and a ready sense of the ridiculous. She travelled daily, with her sister, who was a senior student, from a small town thirty miles north of Salford. Fiona was a keen horsewoman and rose early to exercise her horses before setting off to catch the Manchester train. She had originally wanted to be a vet and had been awarded a place at a prestigious Scottish university, but as all places for women were filled for the next four years, she was informed, she decided to fill in the time by joining her sister in studying physiotherapy – obviously well before equal opportunities.

If ever there was a physio who knocked on the head that we physios were all natural game players, it was Fiona. Just to watch her try to catch a ball in the early days was enough to send us into hysterics. 'You need some intensive training yourself before claiming to teach co-ordination through ball games' our gym instructor remarked drily as she observed her initial pathetic efforts the first week. I suppose in many ways we were opposites, I was fair as she was dark. I was tall and slim while she was of a build straight out of Renoir. Fiona was a Catholic, I was a Quaker and although a great horse rider, she was definitely non athletic where I had been a junior sprint champion and loved sport. Yet in spite of these variances or perhaps because of them, we seemed to get on well together.

In our wider circle of friends were Barbara, Sylvia and Paula. Barbara and Sylvia came from County Durham and Paula from the Lake District. Unlike us, these three lived in digs, at least they did at first but it didn't work out so they moved into the YWCA. Their hostel was in the Whalley Range district of Manchester; perhaps not the most desirable area in those days but it was handy for the Medical school and the teaching hospitals. Anyway as it transpired it was an ill wind…

They were returning home from an outing to the cinema one night when Barbara stumbled over something. Substantially built Barbara landed awkwardly on a partially filled plastic bag. 'Are you alright' enquired her two friends. Barbara replied 'she thought that she was but was sitting on something mighty hard.' As she spoke she dragged from under her ample behind what seemed to be a parcel wrapped in a plastic carrier bag.

'What are you doing with that, throw it away at once,' said Sylvia with obvious distaste, as Barbara began to look in the bag.

'Hang on' said Barbara, 'there is something here that we need, I'm taking it back to the hostel to have a good look.'

With that and much to the distaste of Paula and Sylvia, Barbara marched off refusing to say what she had found. Back at the hostel, Barbara tipped the contents of the bag onto the bedroom floor. 'There what did I tell you' said the triumphant Barbara to her horror struck friends. Lying on the floor was an almost complete collection, of human bones.

'What shall we do with them,' said Paula.

'Do with them,' said the matter of fact Barbara, 'we will clean them up and use them silly, they have obviously come from a skeleton. Look there is no tissue on them.' 'I bet some drunken medical student dropped them on the way home from the student union.'

Next morning, the three bounded into the common room full of the news of their lucky find. By then even Sylvia and Paula were convinced it was a stroke of good fortune. Didn't you consider reporting your find? I had asked tentatively not wanting to sound like a wet blanket. 'You must be kidding,' Barbara had replied, 'it's a skeleton not a body and we are not going to look a gift horse in the mouth.' The three girls enthusiastically described to the rest of the set how they had scrubbed the grubby bones clean and as physiotherapy students, rejoiced in the fact they now had their own almost complete set of bones to help with their studies.

We, who had acquired this costly item by more orthodox means knew the financial saving it was to them and rejoiced at their good fortune.

CHAPTER FOUR

Strangeways and All That

We were just beginning to find our feet in the Physiotherapy School when Bo announced we were to do our two-weeks nursing and that we would find which ward that we had been allocated to, on the notice board. I was to work on the female orthopaedic ward.

The ward had twenty beds, a row down each wall. Most of the beds seem to have all sorts of gadgets and frames attached, both to the bed and to the patient. The patients were mostly elderly with fractured femurs but there were patients that had been involved in road accidents and a few young patients who had congenital problems that required surgery and subsequent fixation. At the end of the ward were the bathrooms and the sluice room which was used for emptying and washing bedpans, rolling washed, dried crepe bandages and packing metal drums with dressings prior to them being sterilised.

'Good morning,' said Sister Jones on my first day. It was nine o'clock and she had been on duty for the last hour and a half. 'You had better start with doing the flowers, you will find them in the sluice. When you have finished come and find me.' I dutifully went to the sluice, and found numerous and varied vases containing mostly chrysanthemums, in varying states of health. Flowers were the staffs' nightmare, they had to be taken out at night because it was thought that they emitted carbon dioxide and brought back next day to patients' lockers for which there was barely room. Because it was such a busy ward, the water in the flowers was rarely changed. At first I washed the vases and tried to arrange the flowers but there were so many, I gave up and just changed the water and popped the flowers back. I loaded the vases onto the trolley and distributed them around the ward as best I could. Even now, although a keen gardener, chrysanthemums are not my favourite flower.

'Next job,' Sister briskly told me, 'was to collect and clean all the dentures from patients who could not do that for themselves.' Oh golly I thought, if anything in this world makes me feel sick it's the thought of false teeth. Steeling myself I took a tray and duly collected all the pots containing the teeth. There, alone in the sluice, quietly heaving up, as my stomach churned, I tried to clean the seven or eight pairs of dentures at arm's length, often with my eyes closed. As I finished each set, I gingerly replaced the teeth into the newly cleaned stainless steel gallipots. As the little lids of the pots snapped close, I breathed deeply glad I had finished. I loaded the pots onto a tray and headed off. As I stepped into the ward, it hit me like a clap of thunder, the pots were not named and did not have bed numbers on them. I had seven sets of teeth and I no idea to whom they belonged. There I stood pole axed trying to decide what to do.

'What did you do,' said Fiona laughing as we compared notes after the first day on the wards.

'What could I do,' I bleated 'I just left a pot on each locker and disappeared to the laundry.'

Nobody seemed to complain except one patient, a couple of days later, when she informed me that when she left she would have to have her dentures seen to.

Over the next two weeks I learned how to become invisible during Matrons ward rounds, make beds with hospital corners and check for nits using carbolic solution and a steel comb.

Salford Royal was our base in the first few months. It was here we treated our first real patients and it was from here that we joined other students for lectures at the Medical School in Manchester.

Our common room, like the casualty department, was in the basement, in fact a considerable portion of the old Salford Royal seemed to be subterranean. The common room was also our changing room and we were always changing. Out of mufti into white coats, out of these into navy shorts and shirts, out of gym kit into less, often much less and so it went on or off, as the case may be.

For our own fitness and teaching sessions, we used Salford's Adelphi Lads' Club. This large community centre was built with money from Salford City benefactors in 1903, who were only too aware of the great poverty in the area, and it was opened by the Chief Scout Baden Powell in 1904. It is in the heartland of industrial Salford and originally built especially for the deprived boys and men of the area. It took us only a few moments to get there. It was out through the back of the hospital with the smell of the nearby large soap factory scenting the air. We ran past the small discretely placed Church Inn, which was hidden behind the large Roman Catholic Cathedral, at least most of us did most of the time. Some male members of the hospital staff, including one or two of our male students, sometimes called in at 'church,' as they put it so as not to alarm patients, for a 'swift half.' Down the narrow cobbled street, lined with the tiny, soot blackened terraces from which most of our patients came. The 'two-up and two-down' houses had one cold tap each and were lit by gas brackets, downstairs only, this, when the rest of the nation had bathrooms and electric lighting. In prolonged spells of bitter weather, these taps would freeze leaving the unfortunate folk, having to resort to the one street tap provided by the 'Corporation.' As we ran past the grim, dark, pawn-cum-second-hand shops, full of dusty, ancient shoes and sad rumpled men's suits, I often wondered what the locals thought of us as we dashed along in our shirt and shorts in the depth of winter. I never remember feeling cold but I certainly remember my chilblains. I always had chilblains.

Our first contact with real patients came with a visit to one of the outpatient clinics. This particular clinic, to which we were being shepherded, was full of veterans, regular customers who eyed us with disconcerting relish. Who was going to treat whom, I wondered. Here because it was a teaching hospital, some patients were allowed to come for extended treatment, dependent on waiting lists and student need. They were all suffering from classic, long term, conditions such as arthritic knees, strokes, chronic bronchitis. These good people knew that not a lot more could be done for them but they came cheerfully as an alternative to being housebound. Even this unpretentious outing gave them chance to socialise. In short we were being let loose on very experienced patients and it was with their heartening compliance we first laid our healing hands on the suffering public.

As these patients were highly experienced, they were expert in their own pathology, treatment and prognosis. They were receptive to new ideas for the most part but it was a wise student who listened to their patients for although most were willing to try anything new, with their experience, they could see the pitfalls, which we, the green and unwary, could not foresee.

As students, we were divided up into small groups and sent to various clinics and departments. Sylvia, Barbara and Paula, found themselves allocated to the Electrotherapy Department amidst a bewildering array of machines for heating, sterilising instruments, vibrating and stimulating weakened muscles. 'There was ultra sound this, ultrasonic that not to mention ultra-violet and infra-red therapy,' moaned Paula.'I hope I didn't cook anyone with those square pulses and sine curves' Paula said.

'You didn't actually treat anyone did you?' I asked.

'We did,' said Sylvia but it was only warm wax therapy we couldn't go far wrong with that, what have you been doing?

'Fiona and I have been to the Plaster room in the Fracture clinic, just to observe.' I said. 'There is a remarkable porter called Tommy who seems to run the place although technically under the supervision of Plaster Sister but it is pretty obvious who really is in charge. Apparently he learned his plaster and splint making skills in the army years ago and those two young housemen check everything with him, before they let the patients go.'

A few days later, I was in one of the treatment clinics having been given a short list of patients to treat. There always seemed to be miscellaneous people hanging about and today was no exception. Feeling a little bit confident, I approached a group of these waiting extras. Trying to sound professional, I enquired if they were being attended to.' They gave me a knowing smile and replied 'that they were waiting for someone.' I turned away puzzled and went over to the Superintendent, as the head of department was then called. 'Those chaps say they are waiting for someone.'

'It's alright,' said the genial plump head of department, 'they are warders from Strangeways prison. They are often here bringing prisoners who come for treatment, you'll soon learn to spot them.'

'I didn't realise we had prisoners' I said interestedly, turning to look round the department, 'what's wrong with them?'

'Oh anything and everything,' said the ever pleasant Miss Hay, 'once inside, any condition under the sun becomes acute, flat feet, bunions, fibrositis. We once had a prisoner who swallowed a lavatory chain pull and all. You see,' she continued 'time spent in hospital is counted as time served that's why some go to bizarre lengths to come here.' I was just digesting this fascinating bit of information when Miss Hay pointed to the three people at the doorway saying, 'here's one of your patients now, the other two are her warders.'

For a moment I stood transfixed. I had only just been slowly assimilating the idea of male prisoners; it certainly had not occurred to me there would be females too. My heart sank – the poor soul. I collected her treatment card and approached the waiting women, 'Mrs Slater' I enquired. One of the women nodded, 'this way please' I said feeling embarrassed by her apparent non-civilian status. Mrs Slater stood up and followed me into the treatment cubicle and took off her coat. It was immediately obvious that she was from the prison. She was wearing, like all the inmates then, the shapeless, blue and white striped, heavy cotton dress. I tried not to stare but before I could avert my eyes from the apparition before me she had caught my glance and I felt her stinging humiliation. The male prisoners wore shirts of the same material and dungarees but as many of our patients came from the docks, factories or pits, wearing pretty much the same sort of work clothes, they did not look too conspicuous at all.

Mrs Slater certainly had flat feet, not the worst I have ever seen but never before or since, have I given such meticulous treatment to the transverse and longitudinal arches of the feet. Occasionally, the prison escort would come and look pointedly at their watch and ask, 'if Slater was ready yet?' I chatted to my patient about things in general but not what she was in for. She knew perfectly well that I was spinning out her treatment time and was grateful for that. It was the prison garb that got to me. Eventually, women were moved out to a prison in pleasant Cheshire where they were able to wear and look after their own clothes, thus saving us tax-payer's money if nothing else.

Being where it was, Salford Royal hospital was not only handy for Strangeways prison but it was nearby to factories, mills, coal mines and the docks on the Manchester Ship Canal which linked the city to the coast at Liverpool. My next patient that morning was Mr Amery who was looking particularly unhappy. Mr Amery had received a nasty injury to his shoulder at work, on the docks and still had very limited range of movement, in fact no more than thirty painful degrees from his side.

'Hello, Mr Amery, what's up?' I asked as I invited him in for treatment.

'I've been to see the doctor in outpatients, seems he had just heard about the Dockers strike and told me to come back when the strike was over.'

I could hardly believe what I was hearing, it seemed incredible that anyone could refuse treating a patient on such grounds. It was the first and only time, I have known that happen but not the only time I have known a consultant play God.

'Come on,' I said trying to cheer him up, 'I'll lay my healing hands on you.' He grinned, knowing full well that the next half hour was going to be no picnic.

CHAPTER FIVE

Trip To The Theatre

It wasn't long before we were told we would be expected to observe in theatre. It was left to us to decide which operations we thought might be of interest to us and then get the necessary permission from the Consultant and inform the all-important Theatre Sister. We would, we were told, be able to find what was on in theatre by checking the daily theatre list in the corridor of the theatre suite.

Fiona and I strolled over to the theatre block one morning debating whether we should spend our first morning in the thoracic or orthopaedic theatres only to find ourselves not alone in checking the theatre lists. As we approached, we saw two patients, complete in dressing gowns, eagerly pouring over the lists of names. It was clear they were acting as the bearers of surgical tidings, good or bad, for their fellow patients.

'Good heavens,' said Fiona 'just look at those two, they look like punters studying the racing Gazette.'

As we approached the notice board the two men moved off, the one in the full leg plaster muttering as they did so, 'I'll tell 'arry he's for the chop tommora!'

'I only hope they have the right Harry,' I whispered to my friend.

Soon after the theatre list was moved to a more discrete place because it was rumoured that a patient had informed his mate that he was for open heart surgery when in fact, he had been admitted for the removal of a benign cyst. The poor patient took these tidings hard, suffered a stroke and his fortune-teller ward mate, an early discharge.

As I was soon to start work in orthopaedic wards shortly, I elected to observe the mid-thigh amputation scheduled first thing the next day. The Consultant performing the surgery was a genial, sturdily built, middle aged man with ginger hair that stood up in short spikes on top of his bullet shaped head.

I duly presented myself, complete in gown mask and boots, wondering if

I too would faint and drop like a stone at the sight of the first incision as so many students are reported to do. The patient, a young man in his twenties, was wheeled in, unconscious. He had cancer in his tibia and amputation was imperative. He was lifted onto the theatre table and his leg swabbed with iodine, the brown liquid running in streaks along his pale skin. Green theatre sheets were placed over him, so soon the only exposed area was an inch of mid-thigh. Totally isolated in this way, the few inches visible could have been anything anywhere. The anaesthetist was sitting at the patient's head, his left hand cupping the patients chin, the right hand busy adjusting the various controls at his side.

'Right ho let's make a start' said Mr Joyce then turning to me said, 'you had better stand here if you are to see anything.' I moved closer and watched in fascination as the smooth skin was slit. The wound edges recoiled as the skin tension was released and blood poured and was mopped up expertly by the nurse whilst the blood vessels were cauterised. After the first shock I watched totally absorbed. The muscles were cut low down near the knee and detached from the bone. The bone was then sawn through higher up. The surgeon holding the flap of muscle moulded a firm pad over the end of the bone and secured the whole stump into a neat package, stitching the skin firmly to ensure the muscle pad covering the bone stayed in place. 'There we are' said Mr Joyce, 'with firm bandaging to ensure a good shape for his 'bucket top,' he will be in your hands in no time.'

Just then, the offending, detached leg, which had been placed in an inadequate bucket, fell over with a sickening crash. 'That was definitely the worst part of the morning, seeing that grotesque mutilated leg, lying there,' I admitted to Fiona later when we were comparing notes. 'It was to go to the medical school for research.'

Arriving at the entrance to the orthopaedic ward the following day, I was met by the physiotherapist in charge, Heather Smith.

'Hello,' she said in an encouraging manner, 'here are your patients' treatment cards, the case notes and x-rays are over there. Bye the way, don't stand any nonsense from Charlie Wood, he's the fractured tibia. I'll be back in half an hour to see how you are getting on.'

Up until now, it had not occurred to me most orthopaedic patients were not ill like those on the thoracic unit or general surgical wards, on being admitted. Yes they are feeling sore, dazed and generally knocked about a bit but they are basically well, coming into hospital as the result of an accident of some sort whether it is on the playing field, in the home or on the road. They have not been deteriorating for some time with a bad heart or galloping consumption.

What is more these fit patients, often young men have to be immobilised for some time and any female under the age of a hundred entering the ward, will be treated as fair game. If you happen to be an eighteen year, old female, so much the better, or worse, depending on whose side you were on.

So unsuspectingly, I made my first mistake by not checking which bed Charlie was in. Like a lamb to the slaughter, I asked for Mr Wood. Several volunteers shouted out all trying to convince me they were Mr Wood. Ignoring all the advice that was coming thick and fast across the ward, I tracked Charlie Wood down. Trying to assume indifference I certainly did not feel, I ignored the whoops, cheers, and whistles, and briskly drew the curtains around his bed. Then in what I hoped was a confident, professional tone I said 'right let's start,' and immediately thought, I could have phrased that better too, but I was getting into my stride and quickly followed it up with, 'show me what exercises you were told to practise.' That was always a good opening gambit, it gave you time to assess the patient and possibly pick the brains of hopefully, a more experienced colleague.

Charlie had stolen a motorcycle, crashed it and, in doing so, fractured his leg, poetic justice but it was a nasty break. As so frequently happens, once isolated behind the screens, away from his mates, the young man was sweetness and light trying to hide his pain when doing his exercises. Even so he reverted to type when I asked him to lift and hold, and there were plenty of stifled sniggers and suggestive comments when I was fool enough to say, 'now resist me,' as I had put my hand firmly on his toes.

I was glad to see Heather on her return and to share the banter. As we left to get a well, earned cup of coffee she said 'I would get used to it. It is all in the tone of voice and terminology. For example you should never say 'open your legs,' always 'separate your feet' – little things like that save a lot of pitfalls.' I nodded how right she was.

After my coffee break, I returned to the ward to see how Eddie, the mid-thigh amputation from yesterday, was. As I walked into the ward I saw a senior physio was treating him. 'Hello,' she said, 'I'm Molly and you are just what we need isn't she Eddie.' Eddie seemed surprisingly cheerful considering all things and I was glad to help and learn. 'First though we must finish your exercises so you can practise when we have gone.' She talked us through her work explaining that having lost most of his leg there would be some twenty per cent body weight loss, which Eddie would not realise until he stood up, so he would have to learn a new balance mechanism. What's more she went on, the powerful hip flexors will try to force the stump up because there is no leg weight to counter them, which is disastrous if he is to wear a prosthesis and walk again. 'So you must do your gluteal exercises as often as possible Eddie, it is vital,' she said patting his backside.

We had Eddie sitting on the side of the bed waiting for his head to clear. Molly asked if he had his shoes with him? 'I might have,' he replied, 'but I definitely have slippers.' Molly looked into his locker and found a shoe.

'Here we are,' then, over her shoulder she said to me 'we never teach walking in slippers, there's no support and they are dangerous.'

'The funny thing is,' said Eddie, 'that I'm getting awful pain in the foot that has gone.'

'It's called phantom foot pain,' said Molly, 'it happens frequently and is caused by the nerve supply to your foot still being intact above the operation site, the pain will go in time.' With that we gave Eddie his crutches and with a firm hand on each side of him we stood him up. He was about to keel over and would have done had both of us not been trained to hold and support him. 'Take some deep breaths,' said Molly.

'I'm OK,' said Eddie, 'what do you want me to do now?'

'Just stand and tighten your gluteals and remember your quads in the good leg, they hold you up' said Molly her hand on Eddies back to encourage him to stand upright.

'You have done very well for first time up,' said Molly encouragingly, as we helped Eddie back into bed. 'We will have another go this afternoon, things will be better then, you will see.' Eddie smiled wanly.

We walked down the ward and Molly thanked me for helping her but really I should have thanked her, I had learned more in half hour than ever I could from two hours with a textbook.

CHAPTER SIX

What Modesty: Shock Treatment

After working with patients for some time, you forget the natural embarrassment people have when they are asked to strip. Not so the hapless physio student who happens to be in the wrong place at the wrong time.

My friends and I were sitting in the common room, when a senior physio walked in. Without any explanation we were told to change into our gym kit and to report to the medical gym at once. Without saying another word she left, leaving us wondering what we were in for?

Suitable attired in our rarely, if ever, washed gym kit, we reported as instructed. We were practically pounced on by Bo who said in a stern voice, 'strip to bra and pants, one to two senior students.' Doing meekly as bidden, we allowed ourselves to be allocated as requested. We were to be guinea pigs for the mock final examinations next month.

'Oh God,' muttered ample Barbara, 'I have a damn big safety pin holding up my bra and worse I'm wearing pink pants, they might have warned us, stand by for the wrath of the Almighty.'

I found myself standing in the corner of the gym trying to look unconcerned as the two senior students eyed me critically. I could see them working through the basic routine. Was my head 'set' straight on my neck, if not why not? Under this intense scrutiny, I tried to adjust my apparent abnormalities. 'Now then stand naturally! Don't take any notice of us,' said one, of my seemingly warped body. I stood there miserable as sin not daring to look round to see how my friends were faring.

The two seniors were furiously writing notes, glancing at me as they debated a point. Finally they circled me twice, walking round first one way then the other until I had the distinct feeling I was taking part in the opening scene from Macbeth.

Abruptly they stopped and told me to lie down on the plinth for the next stage. Palpation, oh Lord. Desperately trying to look unconcerned, I was pushed, prodded and poked. I was measured and weighed. Every bit of my sorely tried body was put through its full range of movement and the results duly noted. I was dying to know if my friends were being meted out the same treatment and in particular how the 'safety pin bedecked,' Barbara was faring. I was out of luck every time I moved the least bit there was Bo hand in her belt face twitching.

Then came the final indignity, the marking in the anatomical landmarks. I lay there transfixed, wishing I had been more generously endowed, chest wise and I had shaved my legs. Eventually I was allowed to stand up. I looked as if I'd had a bad night at the tattoo parlour. There were my red major arterial vessels painted in alongside the blue large ascending veins with the major nerves supplies marked out in bright yellow over all. Standing there, I glumly wondered how long it would take to wash that lot off so that I could travel on public transport without being 'run in.' Suddenly Bo terminated the session. With relief I turned to my friends, we all grinned at one another there was not anything else to do. It looked like a bizarre Maori pageant

As we gathered up our things, Barbara, who was substantially built and refreshingly matter of fact, announced that apparently she had one bosom larger than the other. We stared at her naked upper torso with considerable interest, she seemed equally ample and we told her so. Well that is a relief, I was beginning to feel some kind of freak and with that she put on her bra, hoicking up her abundant gifts of nature and securing the load with her huge safety pin.

The next day, as Fiona and I were walking to the electrotherapy department, my friend was in a considerable state of agitation. It was to be our first practical electrotherapy session and of course that meant practising on each other first. 'I am not, definitely not going to have either faradism or galvanism, I don't mind anything else but I am not going to have either of them.' These currents were used to test damaged muscles and so it was imperative we tried them on ourselves first. Fiona kept up with her protestations.

'Yes, I would have ultrasound which you do not feel or infra-red treatment which was nice and warm, but no electric-shock treatments.' The more she gabbled on the more reassured I felt. Fiona might have been hapless at ball games initially, and was at panic stations at the thought of electric-shock treatments but she was the most feminine girl in our set and without doubt the most academically able. This last gift she put down to the fact her convent school had been an exam factory. She was that rare person who did not seem to work at all yet she must have done. She was widely read on any and all subjects and as she once told me, 'I can't bear not to know.' Fiona was good for me, for unwittingly she showed me it was better to keep up with work rather than be caught on the hop with a spot exam.

I listened to Fiona gabbling away reaching near hysteria, as we approached the 'electro' department. I found it quite comforting to know that she had some weaknesses too.

'It will be all right,' I tried to reassure her for the umpteenth time, 'I'll have both the faradism and galvanic treatment.' However, in her terrified state she seemed totally deaf. I was not feeling all that tranquil either but I kept telling myself it could not be all that bad if we give it to patients.

We entered the department and were met by Mr Petrie. He was middle aged, of medium height and medium colouring. He wore thick tortoiseshell glasses and never raised his voice. He was the sort of person you could see but not describe moments later, in fact a dead ringer for the Secret Service, before the days of James Bond, I had said to Fiona. We were to find out that although he was not the 007 type, he was a patient, conscientious and a very knowledgeable lecturer.

Directing us over to the various pieces of apparatus, we were given an imaginary condition to treat. I was to be suffering from a fractured elbow with nerve involvement with one part of my hand having only partial movement. 'Find out if the nerve is partially damaged or completely ruptured?' asked Mr Petrie. He then added, 'that means using both kinds of electrical current would you not agree?' Fiona nodded with a shade too much enthusiasm. Sitting down resignedly, I presented my arm for treatment.

'Right here goes,' said Fiona wetting my arm to lower resistance to the current. Theoretically she was supposed to try the current on herself first but Fiona was having none of that. 'Just let me know when you can feel anything?' She asked switching on. 'Can't you feel anything at all?' Asked Fiona anxiously. I answered no reluctantly, in case she increased the current strength.

Suddenly my thumb did the most spectacular manoeuvre, it wound upwards and backwards.

'That's it!' we both shouted, '*abductor pollicis longus*.' We were off, there was no stopping us now.

Seeing our jubilation, Mr Petrie came over to see our success. 'That is very good,' he said, his slow smile showing a perfect set of teeth. 'Now change over Miss Gilway you have a tear to your quadriceps tendon, you need faradism.' I watched Fiona go a lighter shade of pale as she unhitched me from the apparatus.

'I am not having any faradism and that is that!' Her voice squeaked as she plumped down on the edge of the plinth. Muttering, she slowly took off her socks and pumps. Taking no notice of her protestations, I continued to collect the necessary bowl of water, pads, electrodes and the rubber strap, the latter not to hit my friend with but to unite Fiona firmly, with the apparatus. Well that is everything I told myself now to deal with Fiona.

Unfortunately for my panicky friend, Mr Petrie stationed himself at the end of the plinth and judging from his benign smile and placid stance he was in no hurry to move off. Perhaps I thought, he had met the 'Fiona syndrome,' before and was rather more alert than his inscrutable countenance portrayed. Taking full advantage of his presence, I grabbed a stool and sitting down facing Fiona, slapped on the wet pad then the electrodes and secured the lot over her mid-thigh with the rubber strap.

'I am switching on now tell me when you can feel anything' I said, avoiding her meaningful look.

'You had better relax that thigh unless you need more current than is necessary Miss Gilway,' Mr Petrie instructed. Fiona's quadriceps slackened abruptly. I had my hand resting over the pad on her thigh and therefore I was part of the electrical circuit. Gradually I turned up the current, and I heard a strangled 'ahg.' I knew I was not hurting her, far from it, after all I could feel the current too. I began to feel much more confident and turned up the current, then, as I moved the electrode about, I was able to make each muscle in the quadriceps group stand out. For Mr Petrie's benefit I named each muscle as I picked it out.

'Well done,' he nodded and with a glance at Fiona he moved away. While my now euphoric friend said exasperatingly 'she knew all along it could not be that bad!'

Twice a week we left the hospital to attend the Medical School for lectures in anatomy and physiology. These were mildly interesting. Particularly the work on the cadavers but for the most part the lecturer was a very poor second to our own Miss Bently. If medical students were constantly subjected to the leisurely air of learning what we experienced at the university, it was no wonder, physiotherapy students were always first with the answers at the combined teach ins that hospital consultants gave.

After a while I decided I could use my time more profitably studying at home, as the Medical School was on my way, I soon found myself skipping more and more lectures if I knew what the subject of the day was. My friends became more and more suspicious accusing me of working too hard and letting the side down. Coward that I am, I denied doing such a thing but the truth was I could do twice the work in the quiet, comfort of our warm kitchen.

I was lucky enough to have my own skeleton at home, a gift from a family friend who happened to be our GP and as a consequence took a great interest in my studies. Our friend had arrived one day soon after I had started my studies with this oblong wooden box containing a full collection of human bones, it was mine for as long as I needed it with the proviso when I no longer needed it I was to pass it on to another needy student. It was second hand of course, probably having gone through several hands but it was in excellent condition. It is a funny thing studying anatomy from a real human skeleton, as opposed to the more common replicas nowadays. I can't remember giving any thought to the origin of it and the poor soul to whom it once had belonged but then perhaps that was just as well. It always came as a bit of a surprise though, when we had visitors who seemed horror struck as they glimpsed a femur or even worse the skull, which I had put down momentarily.

One day the man from the Pru' called on his annual visit and was invited to sit down. He did so or at least was about to when he glimpsed the skull I had been working on leering out from under the cushion that I had quickly tried to hide it behind. Good God he had said as he jumped up. He watched horror struck as my mother calmly placed the offending item on the piano out of harm's way. Keeping a deadpan expression, my mother offered no explanation as to the bizarre choice of ornaments in her home but said in her gentle attentive manner, 'you were saying?'

Skulls always cause trouble especially when they have to be carried about, they certainly don't fit into a handbag. On one occasion, Barbara had borrowed a skull from the department, which was not strictly allowed. She urgently needed to do some revision at home and having nothing better to wrap it in, she used my newspaper. Hurriedly wrapping the skull into an inelegant parcel, she tucked it under her arm and joined us in the usual frantic rush for the bus. Alas it was pouring down and by the time the bus arrived we were all wet through, Barbara's parcel included. We thought we should climb the bus stairs out of the public gaze, as Barbara tried her best to keep her 'homework,' covered. The bus rambled on, the conductor, obviously a Mancunian, born and bred, calling out the place names at each stop. We left our seats and walked to the top of the stairs as the bus approached the university. 'Owens College, Royal Infirmary, Eye 'ospital,' called the conductor. Suddenly the bus gave a violent lurch precipitating the four of us forward. In an effort to stop herself falling Barbara clutched Paula in front of her and let go of the ill wrapped parcel, which shed its soggy newspaper, bouncing down the metal stairs, landing between the feet of the nonplussed conductor.

There it was, wet and shiny, the stare of the wet, vacant, orbits, being matched by the shocked stare of the alighting passengers. 'I know we're running late but I didn't know we 'ad taken that long,' said the bus guard phlegmatically as he eyed us on the bus platform. Scooping up the article under scrutiny, Barbara wrapped it in her scarf, tucked it under her arm and leapt off the bus with the rest of us following in hot pursuit, the spectacle resembling more like a try at Twickenham than a professional group of Bo's refined young ladies.

While we were still based at Salford Royal, the song 'The Happy Wanderer' was at the top of the pops. Everybody seemed to be singing the catchy song, which had been brought here by an Austrian choir and was first heard in this country, at the Welsh National Eisteddfod. At the same time, our gym instructor seemed keen to put exercises to music particularly the exercises used in the ward classes. I was volunteered. To this end, I staggered off to the ward carrying the record and the cumbersome record player.

Musical exercises had been tried the previous day on the womens' minor gynae ward, with considerable success but it remained to be seen how I would fare on men's surgical.

The Sister, who was quite a tyrant, and her nurses, gathered round to watch the spectacle, which did nothing to reassure me. Ward classes are daunting at the best of times, few patients want to start exercising at nine in the morning and even less, if they are in pain or frightened. Still orders were orders and I had no choice in the matter.

Setting up the record player, I turned to my captive guinea pigs and announced in as bright a voice as I could muster, 'good morning gentlemen, sit away from your pillows, put your newspapers down, your cigarettes out and your radios off.' I walked down the ward as I rattled off my requests, smiling as I did so. Great, it seemed to be working. The men put down their papers, stubbed out their suicidal cigarettes and looked at me expectantly. Losing not one bit of the co-operation I was being given, I quickly put on the *Happy Wanderer* record. The patients really couldn't help themselves the music was so catchy and with very little encouragement, elbows were circled, knees bent and stretched and hands clapped in time to the music. At the chorus, everyone sang at full throttle, aerating their post op lungs as well as any physio could possibly hope for.

The whole session had been a great success and even the Ward Sister seemed impressed and congratulated me. I repeated the performance daily during my four, week stint. The patients changing of course as they were discharged and others admitted. I added to the musical repertoire, with *Roll Out The Barrel*, *Who Were You With Last Night* and *The Lambeth Walk*. Well it takes all sorts...

CHAPTER SEVEN

To Hope

We began to spend more and more time at Hope hospital, a larger teaching hospital in a pleasant residential area of Salford. Hope Hospital, (now the new Salford Royal Hospital) stands in large grounds and was completely different in character from 'The Old Royal.' Its patients reflected the difference too. At Salford our patients consisted of miners, men from the docks, factory and mill workers and of course, Strangeways prisoners. There were also many elderly patients who had lived all their lives in the tiny, sooty houses in the cobbled back streets, who did not want to move away from the familiar and their friends. The young people and newlyweds moved as soon as they could, at least they did until the area was cleared to be replaced with smart housing in the lovely new Developments. However, whatever these Salford Royal patients lacked in material wealth, they more than made up in their cheery fortitude, they were the true 'salt of the earth.'

The much larger teaching hospital at Hope had several specialised departments including a large maternity unit. We students were split into groups and allocated to these specialised departments. The anti-natal and maternity units were popular with all the students and the physios were no exception.

As luck would have it and not without a little connivance, Fiona and I, plus our usual small group of friends, were delegated to the Maternity Unit. Here we observed the miracle of childbirth and the not so wonderful experience of episiotomy. At least one of us blanched at the unexpected sight of scissors being produced and without so much as a 'by your leave,' any explanation or seemingly any anaesthetic, the birth canal wall was snipped a good half an inch. When questioned about this later the Sister replied in a matter-of-fact manner, 'much easier to repair than a jagged tear.' We nodded in agreement but had winced with eye watering sympathy with the mother at the time.

'Off to the theatre at once,' commanded the Ward Sister. 'They are doing a removal of a retained placenta on Mrs Brown and she is on her way to theatre now.' We hurried off, there was not a moment to lose if we were to be gowned up in time. We shed our clothes and put on the theatre gear, which Theatre Sister handed us. The anaesthetist was busy with the unconscious patient and all the staff awaited the surgeon.

The patient was slung up in the inelegant but necessary lithotomy position, her feet supported in stirrups, mercifully dead to world, her top half covered by green theatre sheets. Twenty minutes before, Mrs Brown had given birth to a healthy boy in what had been an uncomplicated birth and requiring only a whiff or two of gas and air. Then trouble loomed when the placenta failed to evacuate and here Mrs Brown was in theatre waiting for manual removal under anaesthetic.

Well it was supposed to be manual but judging by the vocabulary of the surgeon, the placenta had a will of its own and was not going to be removed by hand, wrist or forearm. Only by the time the surgeon was practically on his knees with only the point of his elbow visible from the tail end of Mrs Brown was the stubborn placenta dislodged.

'Yea Gods!' Said Fiona in a strangled whisper, her face the colour of an opal, 'if he had gone much further even her tonsils would have surrendered.'

We spent hours teaching mothers-to-be anti-natal exercises, explaining the various stages of labour as we went along. The 'first timers,' were usually very keen and attended regularly and without doubt the confidence that you instilled just by explaining what to expect and when to expect it, made a huge difference. However we did have a couple of lecturers that seemed to be of the opinion we could teach natural childbirth that was quite pain free as well as a beautiful experience, just through exercise and relaxation. I had my doubts. Everyone knows that parturition is involuntary and will happen whatever. Knowing what to expect, being prepared and practising for the great day, certainly does help and prevents panic stations, that I certainly knew to be true but I could not help feeling that the loosen up, breath, pant and relax brigade were not being completely honest. So in later lectures I always made time during our discussions, to talk about the various forms of analgesia available. It was reassuring to the women to share their concerns with one another. Not just the odd whiff of gas and air, help is at hand ladies but sometimes you just have to ask for it and in good time.

CHAPTER EIGHT

New Lecturer and Don Bradman

About this time a new lecturer joined the staff to teach pathology. Dr Hankinson was a young physician working in the hospital and eagle-eyed Bo had spotted this talented doctor and immediately co-opted him to give a series of lectures. Being healthy, young women, this naturally caused not a little interest. The first lecture was on the composition of blood and diseases associated with it.

He stood in front of the blackboard addressing us, looking, as one drooling female described as quite American with his rimless specs, crew cut and being so tall, in fact this smitten girl went on dreamily 'he looks absolutely super and very kissable.' Fiona and I considered these murmurings and took a critical look at this guy; he hadn't struck us quite so forcibly. We began to study him in minute detail not really listening to what he was saying until he pointedly said to me, 'perhaps you will oblige.' Caught on the hop and before I knew what I was letting myself in for I muttered, 'er yes.' Without more ado, he took a firm hold of my left hand and smartly jabbed my middle finger with a hefty sized weapon, which he laughingly called a needle. Before I could squeak in protest, I had offered my blood up for God, Queen and science not to say for the huge amusement of my colleagues.

Dr Hankinson carefully collected my blood onto a slide to send to the path lab remarking we should have the results back in time for the next lecture. As the learned Dr had predicted he did have the blood results when we saw him again. I discovered my blood group was 'O' positive, that I was hugely anaemic and in need of an intensive course of iron.

Hurrying to Piccadilly later that evening, to catch the bus home, I was caught up by no other than Dr Hankinson. It seemed we were both heading for the same bus. We sat upstairs on the bus chatting and I discovered his home was in Chester but he had a flat in one of the houses overlooking the river Mersey in our district. I knew the houses; they were large elegant Georgian places with huge gardens that rolled down to the river. As the bus rumbled on I thought what a charming and fun guy he was, when suddenly, it was my bus stop. Leaping up and apologising at the same time I said I was about to miss my stop. Excusing my hasty departure, I stood to pass him and head for the stairs, when he asked if I would have dinner with him?

'Yes, thank you,' I gabbled.

'But I don't know where you live?' He called

I gave him the first thing to hand, my library ticket, which was in my pocket. 'Here's my card' I said, leaping off the already moving bus. With 'I will call for you at seven,' ringing in my ears, I fairly skipped home.

For the last six weeks I had been going out with a handsome tall Greek student whom I had met at a university hop. He was quiet, polite, shy and a wonderful dancer. His smile lit up as I suddenly grasped the required movements of the rumba and from then on there was no stopping us as we chasséd across the dance floor every Saturday night for the next few weeks. As the days progressed to the end of term he asked me if I would attend his graduation as his family lived in Ethiopia. I said I would and did, celebrating afterwards with dinner. We both knew that nothing would come from our friendship but it was very pleasant while it lasted.

The next day armed with his accountancy degree he flew to Athens to visit friends and relatives, on route for Ethiopia. There, in Addis Ababa, he re-joined his family and in particular his father's Company.

My parents had been a bit worried by this friendship I could tell. They of course did not say as much to me but I felt their unspoken fear that I might be contemplating married life in 'inconvenient,' Ethiopia.

So it was with the certain knowledge that practically any Englishman, let alone a very presentable one like John, would be made extra welcome in my parents' home that night, I informed my mother I would not be in to dinner. My mother barely disguised her relief with happy curiosity as she remarked I had not wasted much time.

John called for me promptly at seven and as I introduced him to my parents, I knew they approved and I was happy for them. Predictably everything was done properly, the dinner, the wine just right and the whole evening rounded off by a romantic stroll by the river back to my home. As I climbed into bed, I wondered if I would tell my friends at the hospital. Perhaps, perhaps not, in fact I only told Fiona, I knew my secret was safe with her and we both enjoyed the continuing mooning of the besotted student who had no idea of my involvement.

One evening when we were out together, John announced that as he was not on duty the following day and he was going to Old Trafford to see the

Test Match. It was a pity I could not go with him too, 'the weather promises to be great.' I replied that I would go. John looked both shocked and amused so I tried to justify my proposed truancy.

'Look,' I said, 'I have never had a day off from the hospital, in my life and considering that all treatments are given by unpaid students, the paid staff might like a turn.' Then I added emphatically, 'anyway, I'm coming with you.'

'Well I can see you have made up your mind, I'll see you at ten o'clock then.' He smiled, 'I look forward to tomorrow.'

As planned, we met at ten o'clock and caught the bus to Oxford Road station, where we took the train the short distance to Old Trafford cricket ground. It promised to be a gloriously sunny day later in the morning but as we entered the grounds amongst the massing cricket enthusiasts, there was a thin haze overhead. We sat down on a rug that John had thoughtfully brought, it was long before the grassy banks surrounding the outfield were converted to seating areas. John obviously had timed our arrival, perfectly; soon the ground was packed out. It was surprising how many of the public were on holiday considering it was midweek. As expected, Don Bradman made his century. I distinctly remember being helped to my feet, to join everyone else in the late afternoon, to clap the hero back to the pavilion. It had been the most super day.

We took the train back to where we were going to catch our bus. At the bus stop, it must have been obvious where we had been because the men in the bus queue asked John about the match and what the latest score was. I just wondered how I could explain my sunburn the next day.

It had been a memorable day. John and I continued to go out together occasionally over the next two or three years, I continuing with my studies, he, working in different hospitals before moving down to London. Eventually John went to America where he probably still is, America's gain and our loss.

CHAPTER NINE

Ward Classes

If, as students, the ward classes at Salford Royal filled us with holy terror, then we were in for a nasty surprise. The seemingly inappropriately named Hope Hospital had enormous wards and the male orthopaedic ward was no exception. All too soon it was my turn to work on that unit and primed by graphic warnings from those who had gone before, I went forth with all the enthusiasm of the condemned.

There were thirty fit fellows enjoying their very own sport of baiting the next female to enter the ward; yes it had a charm all of its own, first thing on a Monday morning. Like all forms of class taking, the teacher stands or falls by their approach and entry in the first minute or so, and ward classes for the physiotherapist were no exception. There needed to be just the correct balance of cheerfulness and authority to get any co-operation what so ever. So, with the well-rehearsed 'good morning gentlemen, please sit up, put your radios off, your newspaper down and your cigarettes out,' I made my opening gambit. Having gained their attention thus far, I walked up and down the ward with what I hoped was a purposeful tread, extolling these young athletic types to do their exercises.

Wearing my cloth ears to the odd, often very odd, bawdy remark and keeping a beady eye on the ward comedian, I moved along the feet of the regimented beds. So far so good, I told myself, then suddenly there was something cold and wet running down the back of my legs. I spun round, Ginger Jones, the fractured patella, was earnestly doing his exercises, looking as if butter would not melt in his mouth. I must be mistaken I thought or rather hoped, as I tried to keep the momentum going. Down the ward I went with an encouraging smile to Derek, the TB spine lying in his plaster of Paris shell bed, doing his restricted best with the exercises. Back up the ward, pausing to check Mr Burgess, multiple fractures from Saturday night and yes, there it was again, cold wet down the back of my legs. I whirled round, Ginger Jones again, looking all too innocent, why had I turned my back on him? As the cold rivulet ran down the back of my legs I could hear the muffled sniggers in the ward. With what I hoped was remarkable aplomb, I kept going, then suddenly spun round and caught the wretched Ginger Jones nicely. He was busy loading a water pistol from the vase of daffodils on his locker. Giving him a purposeful look as I walked over to him, I pocketed the water pistol and promised I would be back.

The ward class finished uneventfully and I went over to the luckless Ginger and drew the curtains around his bed, probably more slowly than usual. Telling, the now worried, red-head to take off his pyjamas, as he might as well have his individual treatment now. For the next ten minutes he sweated and moaned and sweated and muttered 'bloody ell' as his physiotherapist carefully put him through his post-op routine. It was a very subdued Ginger I left as I drew back the curtains and he scrabbled to cover himself up.

CHAPTER TEN

Nightmare

After eighteen months the first major external examinations loomed large on the horizon. The external exams were to be taken at a teaching hospital, chosen by The Chartered Society of Physiotherapy. In theory the exams could be taken anywhere in the UK, in practise they were held at the nearest School of Physiotherapy.

This first hurdle in our career consisted of three written papers, Anatomy, Physiology and Electro-mechanics, followed by two vivas, oral examinations. Every exam segment had to be passed before we could proceed to the next stage of our professional career. For me personally, this was the great test. I had to admit that as reluctant as I had been to re-join the world of physiotherapy, I found myself enjoying both the theory, and the practical work with the patients and of course I had made new friends too.

Night after night found me at home in the comfy kitchen, my feet tucked cosily beside the always warm range. Here I would expound out loud to an imaginary examiner, the compulsory detail required. I would hold forth on everything from individual muscles to inter-tissual fluid or the medulla oblongata. Talking out loud in this way helped me to remember tedious detail. When trying to remember something I could hear my voice speaking in my mind eye as it were.

Over the weeks I worked systematically, literally from head to toe, trying to learn and talk about everything in between and inclusive. Now and again I was swamped by the enormity of the task and was only too glad that from the beginning I had tried to keep abreast of the work. That, I found was the only way I could do my work. For me cramming at the last moment is not an option. I would go into mental blackout. Further, and probably most important of all, I had promised my father to 'give it a try,' and as reluctant as I was at first, I was surprised that by keeping abreast of my work, I enjoyed it.

The gods must have been with me in this self-imposed, work ethic for two weeks before the exams were due, family tragedy struck.

My father had only two relatives in the whole world other than his immediate family, his younger sister, my Auntie Amy and his mother, my grandmother – both dearly loved. Auntie Amy was slender, elegant, with milk-white skin, dark hair and green eyes and the most perfect set of white teeth I have ever seen. In many ways she was a woman ahead of her time. In her youth my father had taught her short-hand, which he had taught himself earlier, 'just in case it might come in handy.' From somewhat impoverished beginnings, she, through sheer ability and hard work became a company director in a highly profitable organisation. Auntie Amy and my father were very close, the more so because she had never married. She lived with my grandmother, in considerable style.

I never remember either my aunt or my feisty, four foot eight, Yorkshire grandmother, to be ill, ever. One day though, my aunt had persistent aching in her shoulder and went to the doctors. He diagnosed fibrositis and treated for such, all to no avail. The pain grew rapidly worse as did the movement in the shoulder. In sheer desperation, she consulted another local doctor, one who only took private patients. He examined her and told her he would make an appointment to see a consultant up the road. Up the road was 'The Christie,' the famous cancer hospital.

Even with all the expertise this world famous hospital could offer, Auntie Amy was a stricken woman. The malignancy was advanced and already affecting her cervical and brachial plexuses, resulting in great pain and disfiguring paralysis of her face and arm. The disease spread, her facial nerve was destroyed, her mouth sagged and eating and drinking were difficult.

All this time my aunt refused to acknowledge the enemy. She doggedly went to work, driving her car for as long as she was able, never taking painkillers for fear it would confuse her mentally.

Although my parents were aware of the gravity of my aunt's illness, Auntie Amy was insistent her mother should not be told. This caused its own problems, tough grandma was never ill and a great walker. Sometimes when she took us out 'to town,' she would insist on walking home, a five mile journey. If we should so much as moan about getting a bus, she would march us off with a 'don't be so soft,' and that was definitely that. So it was, as my aunt grew more and more tired, my elderly grandmother, not understanding the situation, would tell her in her brusque, Yorkshire way, 'to pull herself together and shape.'

My brave aunt battled on, my parents giving what support they could but Auntie Amy never asked for help, to her it would have meant conceding to the inevitable. Her quiet dignity impressed all, including her new doctor. The

GP was very understanding, supporting her through her ordeal, giving her confidence in him not least by not pretending about how serious things were. He prescribed painkilling drugs although he knew she did not take them. The doctor and my aunt had a pact that reassured her utterly. The pact was that should she need him he would come whatever time of day or night it might be.

So it was that shortly before my exams, one frightful Saturday night, my aunt asked my father to summon the doctor. The situation could not have been more heart-breaking. My father knew exactly what he was being asked to do when he asked the doctor to attend. He knew his beloved sister could not endure any more. She had fought to the last. She had somehow or other dragged herself into work on the Thursday but just couldn't manage Friday. My father totally overcome with a feeling of hopelessness, called the doctor, who true to his word came at once. The doctor went straight to Auntie Amy's room and gave her an injection to relieve her dreadful pain. For the first time in months my aunt was without pain and fell into a peaceful sleep with me sitting by her side. I sat and tended my aunt until she died peacefully three days later, never having regained consciousness.

It was all so devastating. Auntie Amy was the bravest woman I have ever met and we all felt her death hugely. From then on the pattern of our life changed.

Ever since I could remember, we always went to see grandma on Sunday morning after first going to Quaker Meeting. My mother did not go with us rather returning home to prepare Sunday lunch. At grandma's we were always give a warm welcome. She would give us a huge slice of cake, usually ginger cake, my father's favourite and as it was nearing lunchtime, the cake was followed by a substantial dish of delicious creamy rice pudding. We ate all that was put in front us of course, then told to wash our hands before being allowed into the beautifully furnished drawing room. There we would often listen to Auntie Amy sing in her wonderful contralto voice, sitting on the floor 'so as not to untidy the cushions.'

Sitting on the floor was no hardship. There was thick carpet with deep-pile rugs in front of the cosy fire. My father used to joke to us about 'there being such a thing as being too house proud' but we knew this grandma had been born in the Workhouse in the mid-1800s and had endured a hard life, until her children were in a position to alter things. It was just that, what grandma had, was hard won and therefore cherished and even we children fully understood.

As we kissed our grandmother and Auntie Amy goodbye, we would be given our pocket money, mine was less than my elder brother but more than my younger brother. My money was always banked. For the journey home we were given two sweets and often flowers from the garden for my mother.

True to family tradition, my father was also a great walker and thinking that we had better work up an appetite for the Sunday roast my mother always produced, we would walk the three miles back home. I could never understand why my mother bothered, we never could do justice to the laboriously prepared meal. Indeed my poor mother would complain bitterly about us having had our appetite spoilt, on the other hand my father wasn't too popular if, 'we didn't eat up,' at grandma's. Why my mother struggled on over the years, when she could have taken a much needed, rest, I never could understand. Years later whilst the whole family were enjoying a lovely Sunday picnic, I asked my mother why and she laughed and said,

'I don't know, it just was tradition, I must have been mad.'

The whole lifelong pattern of Sundays changed. Grandmother, bereaved, was completely distraught. Now, she was on her own in a large house, nobody to cook and keep house for, nobody coming through the door in the evenings. They had always lived together and now it seemed to her that the very purpose of her life had been snuffed out. It also was an added cruel twist of fate that Auntie Amy had died on grandma's birthday. On every birthday until now, my aunt had arranged a splendid feast for her mother, the grand climax of the party being a huge beautifully decorated ice cream cake which, because it was the days before fridges, was delivered to the door moments before, by 'the man from Walls.' The birthday party was only part of the annual treat. There was just time to wash our hands, and never time to do the washing up, before the taxi arrived. A taxi, we never rode in a taxi, the only means of transport at our house was bus, sometimes train or 'Shank's pony.' There was more, we were on our way to the pantomime in town. Actually, I wasn't very fond of pantomimes with their infuriating way of never getting on with the story and their rude, slapstick sense of humour. But I held my tongue about such trivialities. Who could hate going to a smart theatre in such imperial style, sitting by our regal selves in the Royal Box, sustained by an enormous box of the finest chocolates, the likes of which we rarely saw and certainly never purchased? Even during the interval, our very own waitress brought our own tray of coffee to the royal box and very gratifying it was too, as I imagined the whole world to be watching us.

Yes, everything changed. My grandma became more and more disorientated, managing to lock herself out of her house frequently and unaccountably, yet refusing to allow my father a door key. She began to have mysterious falls for no obvious reason, she who thought nothing of walking the odd-six miles or so. She would forget to put the stopper in her hot water bottle, resulting in mountains of washing.

Things rapidly became worse. My father, trying to fill the void left by Auntie Amy, called on his mother every evening on the way home from work, usually to face a new calamity. At the very least he needed house keys.

At last in sheer desperation, my father sought the help of the GP. The plan was for my father to call on his mother as usual and, while he was there, for the doctor to arrive 'unexpectedly.' The agreed time for this visit was a little later than usual being seven o'clock rather than six. To give a reason for this unusual visiting time, it was agreed I would accompany my father on this tricky mission.

We arrived at the gate a little before seven. The house was in complete darkness. Having no key, my father rang the doorbell then walked round to the back door. There was no reply to our louder and louder knocking. The house stood in disturbing dark silence. We stared through the windows, hesitatingly at first, the curtains were not drawn and we didn't want to frighten my grandmother. The windows seemed to be misted up though we could see the glow of the fire indistinctly. After a while, my now, very anxious father said, 'I'll have to get into the house somehow, I don't like the look of that fire, go to Evelyn's and call the fire brigade, I'll wait here for the doctor.'

I hurried off to our good friend next door to ask if I might use the phone. She asked me in at once seeing my worried face but put her fingers to her lips for me to speak quietly. Evelyn, a teacher, coincidently was unmarried, lived with her elderly mother. They had both been very upset at the death of my aunt and Evelyn was understandably, trying to protect her mother from further distress.

The fire brigade arrived in minutes announcing their arrival with lights flashing and bells clanging. 'Good gracious, mother won't like that,' my father said. With a great squeal the fire engine pulled up at the gate followed by a lesser squeal as the following police car stopped behind it at the same time silencing its siren.

I explained to the leading fireman what the problem was and he at once called for a ladder. Breaking into the lavatory window he came downstairs and opened the front door. My father hurried past him into the kitchen, it was empty except for thick smoke from something that had obviously been grilling for a long time.

My father turned abruptly with me at his shoulder and went back along the hall to the drawing room and opened the door. It was pitch black and smoky with a peculiar smell that caught at the back of our throats. My father groped for the light switch and switched the light on. As the light went on my father cried out in great anguish, turned, and dashed out of the house. Until my father rushed past me, I could not see what had happened, then, it was all too apparent.

There was my grandmother lying headlong in the fire, her head and shoulders completely destroyed by the flicking embers. I stood there riveted to the spot the firemen standing close by me in case I keeled over. I didn't. I stood there taking in the hideous sight. The room was without a sound, the silent, mature, fire glowing bright orange amongst the human cinder in the grate. Stretched out on the once beautiful rug was the rest of my grandmother, small flames lazily licking their way down her body. The only parts unmarked were her legs ending in her beautiful tan leather ankle boots, a Christmas present from her daughter. I seemed to take the whole sight in a flash and realised it was my dearest father that needed my help such as I could give. Then following my father, I bolted from the house. What must he be thinking? Daily, since the death of his sister, he had called to see his mother on the way home from work. Tonight, just to get a house key, he was two hours later, perhaps the difference between life and death. Dear God, how my poor father must be blaming himself.

Thank goodness for Evelyn, there was my father wrapped up in a blanket, sitting in a large armchair by the fire. She was doing her best to keep my father warm but judging by his expression, he was in deep shock. Somehow or other Evelyn, had managed to hurry her mother upstairs to bed, the air so charged with disaster that the elderly lady was getting very agitated.

Then, at last, the doctor arrived. There was obviously nothing he could do for my grandmother so he had been directed to our friend's house where he attended to my father. 'I have to tell my mother what has happened and we are not on the phone,' I said to no one in particular and immediately the doctor offered to drive me the three miles home.

As soon as the car stopped, I leapt out and knocked furiously on the front door. As my mother answered the door, I rushed in with my startled mother hurrying after me. I sagged into the fireside chair and gabbled out what had happened. My elder brother, who had been getting ready to go out, came out of the kitchen and listened, in his hand a newly polished shoe. From the depth of another armchair, my younger brother stared wide eyed, and shivering. The doctor, about whom I had completely forgotten, stood silently in the doorway. Before I could elaborate on any details my mother was putting on her coat and said 'we must go to your father at once.' The doctor, seeing there was nothing more he could do, bade us good night and I showed him to the door, thanking him for his help.

My Brother, Gerald, brought the car to the front door while my mother made arrangements for my younger brother to stay with a neighbour. Soon we were hurrying back to my father, with my elder brother asking me to tell him again exactly what had happened. As I explained he kept saying, 'oh dear, dear.'

The crowd of spectators had mercifully gone as we turned the final corner and my mother hurried off to Evelyn's. My brother and I went to speak to the fire officers and police who were awaiting my return.

Father seemed less shocked when I eventually saw him next, though still understandably, hugely grief stricken. The dreadful torturing thought that if only he had gone directly to his mother's house as usual, things would have been different kept sweeping over him in great unmerciful waves. The doctor had tried to reassure my father his mother had collapsed and died before she had fallen into the fire and having seen the position of grandma and being used to analysing human posture, I felt he was right and told my father so. But for me too, though I would never admit it, there was always the totally hideous thought that she might have lain helpless in the fire. I squeezed my eyes tightly to blank out the terrible thought.

The night continued, my mother returning home with my brother and my father and I going to the police station to make a statement. 'There will have to be an inquest which is held in the Coroners Court, you will be told about it as soon as it can be arranged,' the Sergeant on duty, informed us.

Somehow it was well after midnight as we left the police station. The night air was pleasantly cool and quiet. In the silence, father and I walked together, lost in our thoughts, not talking. A police car drew up alongside and the officer asked us if we would like a lift home. My father, a great walker and now on autopilot said, 'no thank you' at the same time as I said,

'yes please.' I was feeling physically drained and instinctively felt that my father felt the same but would not admit it.

The kindly officer jumped out of the car and helped us into the back seat. He drove us home and we were grateful for the three mile lift and for his understanding silence.

Totally exhausted, the family retired to bed. For me at least, there was to be no sleep. Every time I closed my eyes, the horror of the night flooded in with sharp, crystal clarity, in fact it was worse in the darkness, everything replayed with hideous brilliance. I heard the clock strike four and decided I couldn't stand it any longer. I crept into my parents' room, vaguely thinking that they might like a cup of tea. Instead I found myself saying, as I had when I was a child, 'I can't sleep.' The response from my wide, awake parents, was immediate,

'come and tuck your toes under the eiderdown,' and moving up, made room for me.

So there we were, all snug in the warm bed. There wasn't much room but then there wasn't much left of the night. We derived comfort from our togetherness and instantly we fell into a blissful, deep sleep.

There was an inquest some time later, which we all had to attend. The actual cause of death, could not be accurately ascertained, the charring was too extensive. An 'open verdict,' was recorded.

CHAPTER ELEVEN

First Hurdle

Not surprisingly I was late for work the following morning. I could have had time off but I preferred to go to the hospital. I thought the discipline of the familiar routine might keep my mind off things. I was wrong. The flash backs kept flashing back. I was like a zombie, it was a good job I was attending pre exam lectures and not treating patients.

Unknown to me, my father had phoned Bo before I had a chance to get to the hospital. I called at Bo's office, as a courtesy, to explain my late arrival. She was kindness itself. Gone was the clipped matter of fact tone of speech she usually used as she said, 'Your father has been telling me about the help you were to him last night.'

Surprised and feeling a little disconcerted, I replied truthfully, 'I didn't do much, I was just there.'

'Maybe,' she said and studied me quizzically.

As I left Bo's office, I felt instinctively, that she was seeing me in a new light. I had no idea what my father had said on the phone, he wasn't much for talking about himself and certainly not on the phone. When I returned home that evening, he never told me, but from that time on, I was never the recipient of her famous barbed, comments or her considerable talent for sarcasm. Indeed before I was to qualify, I was to have very real evidence of this newly found confidence in me, on at least two occasions.

It is amazing how having confidence in one, gives one confidence. It was a very pleasant feeling and just then, exactly what I needed.

I joined my colleagues in the lecture theatre. It was good to be back with Fiona. A discussion was taking place on the 'popliteal triangle.' It seemed this area behind the knee had not cropped up in recent exam papers and therefore a question on it seemed highly probable. I tried to set my mind to the task in hand, repeatedly forcing myself to concentrate. There were only three weeks to the exams and that included the Easter break. I had to pass those exams to be able to continue with my studies. I did not want to disappoint my father now of all times, but most of all, I wanted to succeed for me.

I went through the motions the first few days but bit by bit, as I was able to sleep better, my concentration began to return. You never forget such a nightmare but time has allowed me to encompass it.

My mother decided we would go away for the Easter break. We never went away so early in the year but as she said, 'these were exceptional circumstances and a break will do us all good.' We went to Arnside, an area of outstanding natural beauty, where we had previously spent many delightful holidays and nearby where I had been away at school. We loved the area, on the Kent estuary, overlooking the mountains of the Lake District.

We travelled by train, I, staring out of the window for the first few miles, seeing nothing, then I came to and opened the bag I had with me, took out a text book, coloured pencils and paper. I read for a while then taking the pencils and paper, began to draw. Passengers, in the nearby seats tried, to see what I was drawing to no avail, it wasn't recognisable. I screwed up my third sheet of paper and started again, labelling it as I did so. At last I had it right I. I had correctly drawn and labelled the origins and insertions of all the muscles of the face and skull and named their nerve supplies. I put the paper down, that would have to do for now I told myself. A few moments later we drew into the small station and I quickly stuffed my book and papers into my holdall and that's where they remained for the whole of the glorious Easter.

Once again that beautiful, tranquil, corner of England had wrought its magic. I felt so much better as I walked through the hospital doors after Easter The waiting was over.

I entered the common room and there amongst the chattering, panicky candidates sat Fiona. She was quietly reading by herself, even at the eleventh hour and amidst the surrounding Babel, she was able to shut out the world and learn. I envied her that gift.

The next few days passed in an air of unreality. I can't remember the questions but in common with anyone else who has sat important exams, I will remember the invigilator announcing, 'you may begin' and the following momentary inability to focus my eyes on the print.

I do remember the vivas though. Standing outside the examination room waiting for my name to be called then with sickening clarity, I heard, 'Miss Arden.' I entered the room and found myself looking at two vastly different people. One, a woman built like a prop forward, the width of her shoulders only equalled by the depth of her impressive bosom. The other examiner, a weedy looking man with no distinguishing features at all. The large woman commandeered me and walked me to a plinth on which lay a first year student who looked at me with considerable sympathy.

'Turn over,' the examiner barked to the student who quickly rolled over onto her face. Yanking up the student's shirt the examiner said, 'put your finger on the twelve dorsal vertebra.' I counted the spinal processes just to make sure and stopped. 'Describe the structures under your fingers,' she said, her eyes glued to where my hand rested. My mouth went dry then, prodded into action by her, 'I'm waiting,' I started in the tone common to anatomists and undertakers, beginning,

'working from the superficial to the deep, we have the skin, superficial facia.' As I worked deeper and deeper the examiner suddenly stopped me and said,

'Describe the structures under your left hand.' I stared at her, not at first understanding the question; I looked down at my left hand and found I had inadvertently rested it on the students waist and lower ribs. My already dry mouth went even drier as I once again described the structures under my hand, mentally stripping away muscle layers. My monologue was suddenly interrupted with a crisp, 'what is the nerve supply,'

'The lower costal nerves' , I offered.

'Good, thank you Miss Arden,' and with that I was steered over to the door to await my colleague, who had the luck, to have been allocated to the weedy chap in the far corner.

The physiology exam was no better. My name was called and I entered the same room to be met by three people. The first, a Professor Davis asked me, 'what subject would you like to answer questions on?' What should I say, I thought, whatever I say he will think that's my strongest subject and expect great answers? He stood there waiting so I suggested doubtfully,

'the circulation.'

'Right' he said with a suspiciously pleasant approach. For the next ten minutes he tried to tie me up in knots. He succeeded. I left the room having no idea how I had done.

'How did you get on' asked Barbara, who was waiting her turn,

'awful he asked me what I wanted to answer questions on, it threw me a bit.' By this time Sylvia had joined us and stood listening, they could see I didn't want to talk so they didn't press me for more details.

I was going to wait to see how the rest of my friends had faired, but then I thought that might depress me too much. 'I think I will go home, can you tell Fiona I will be in touch.' My friends nodded as I put my coat on. I went home to forget the whole wretched business.

It had been my intention to look around the shops, a rare treat but the closer I walked to the department stores, the more I felt I just could not be bothered. What I needed right now was a good cup of tea, in the swaddling comfort of my own cosy home.

We were given the rest of the week off, after our exams but no more, we had patients to treat. Our results were not due out for a further three weeks but I was determined not to get into pointless discussions about the possible rights and wrongs of the examination questions. What was done was done. I had promised myself I would do all manner of lovely things once the exams were over but somehow it didn't work out like that. I was in mental limbo. The newly found free time was frittered away with no purpose or direction.

CHAPTER TWELVE

Birthday Presents

It had been my birthday a week before my grandmother had died. She and my Auntie Amy had arranged to give me a beautiful gold watch with a lovely delicate bracelet type strap. As my aunt had died six weeks previously, it was with a great deal of emotion that grandma gave me the precious gift. Meanwhile my younger brother was still working on his present for me.

Sometime later, close friends of the family came to visit and one of them asked how I was, meaning how was I coping after the awful trauma of recent weeks. I said truthfully 'that I thought I was doing alright but for one thing.' I admitted going into an empty house was now unpleasant especially in the dark, and worse, as I switched on the light, it triggered a flash back. I hadn't mentioned this to my family, we were all trying to come to terms with recent events, in our own way and I didn't want to cause a fuss. The family friends clucked in sympathy and gave me a hug.

My younger brother, who had been present when our friends had visited, suddenly had a wonderful brainwave and bought me just the right birthday present. A friend of his owned a dog, which had a large litter of puppies and he was finding it difficult to find homes for them. Enter my brother, a man on a mission. My birthday present solved, a puppy's life saved, and I, always had a friendly, noisy, welcome when I entered the house. Perfect, well almost.

The puppy, of doubtful parentage, was short haired, black, white and tan, had floppy ears and an incredibly long tail that everyone said I should have had docked. I didn't. I called my dog Epaminondaas, after the fictional little black boy that was always getting into trouble. Pandy, as he became known, certainly lived up to his original name in the early days. He wet the carpets, dug up all newly planted bedding plants and had an insatiable appetite for the legs of polished furniture.

Worse was to follow as time passed. After a lot of unsubtle hints, I persuaded my elder brother to buy me a pair of black-strapped evening shoes, for the May Ball. 'It was imperative I have them now, so that I have them in time, it will be too late if you wait until my birthday!' I had pleaded. At last he agreed, he gave me the money and off I went and bought the most elegant black evening shoes. I was in Heaven. In my bedroom, I examined my precious shoes and luxuriated in the pleasure of having something that was not purely practical for the first time in my life. I, pirouetted round in front of my long bedroom mirror, yes, they were perfect.

My mother called me to dinner. I reluctantly took off my evening shoes and placed them in their box and went down to join my family. Half an hour later, I went upstairs to look at my beautiful shoes. They were ruined. Lying out of their box, they had hundreds of shiny white teeth marks all over the heels, which had been cut to ribbons. I was distraught. The shoes were the first real luxury that I had ever had. I wanted to weep, there seemed to be no justice in the whole wide world. There was of course no sympathy from my elder brother, quite the contrary. Only my mother remained practical. 'Hand them to me, I'll see what I can do.' My mother had great skill in leather craft and at one time had taught the subject. Ten minutes later she was back. 'There that is the best that I can do.' With a warm iron and a great deal of patience, she had eased the shredded patent leather back into place, smoothing it down. Any white shiny marks, she had coloured in with her Indian ink, she was also a talented artist. I looked at my shoes; they were vastly improved though still marked. 'Nobody is going to look that closely,' added my mother trying to comfort me.

'Anyway,' chipped in my elder brother, 'nobody is going to look at your legs!' I felt like throwing the shoebox at him, my legs were my one claim to fame. I thanked my mother for her efforts and, as she had predicted, no one did notice at the Ball, everyone was busy having too good a time.

Pandy was a highly intelligent dog and as he grew older he calmed down but he did get up to some bizarre pranks. One day I caught him struggling down the pathway with the femur, which I had been studying and had not put away. The bone was as long as himself, but Pandy, wasn't giving up. He determinedly dragged the dry, ancient bone along, doubtless to hide his unwieldy treasure in the recently planted flowerbed. I don't know why he was bothering it couldn't have tasted of anything.

One morning, as I set out to catch my bus to the hospital, I happened to turn round and saw Pandy following me. He must have slipped out of the house as I left. 'Go home,' I said, he stopped and sat down. I hadn't the time to run back and take him home, I just hoped that he would as usual, obey me. It was rush hour, and I was worried. I hurried on then, stopped and turned again; there he was, following me. I told him to go home at once and he stopped in his tracks. I saw my bus coming in the distance as I crossed the road, there was no time to lose or I would be very late. At the same time I saw another bus coming in the opposite direction and it was nearer. Oh goodness I thought I hope he doesn't try to cross the road to catch me up. Then I looked again the bus had stopped opposite me and when it moved off, there was no sign of Pandy. My bus arrived and as I sat down, I pondered the mystery of my disappearing dog. Later, at dinner that night, I was relating all this to my family and my younger brother laughed and said,

'didn't you know, he is always catching the bus, he nips upstairs and hides under the back seat. He was going to see his friend, an old lady across the park and was probably getting anxious about missing his ride when you kept telling him to go home.' I hadn't known about his canine antics but we all laughed as we imagined him getting fed up and nearly missing his bus because of me.

CHAPTER THIRTEEN

Takes All Types

I was back at work the following Monday and my first patient of the day was Mrs Williams who, bless her, was always pleased to see me. She had suffered a stroke, and at the time, had fallen fracturing three ribs and her wrist, 'all on the other side.' It always took me a good half hour to treat Mrs Williams so I heard a great deal about her.

She had left school at the age of ten like many of her classmates, to supplement the meagre family income. The day after leaving school, she started work at the cotton mill, the hours, seven in the morning until six o'clock at night. 'We were woken up at six o'clock, every morning, except Sunday, by Charlie, who used a long bamboo pole to tap on the bedroom window until we called to him. Charlie was our knocker-up and we paid him a few coppers a week. His round consisted of several streets, a bit like the window cleaners today. Sunday, we had an extra hour in bed. At work, the first thing that struck you was the terrible noise, the clackety clack of the machinery and looms and the air was full of cotton dust' said Mrs Williams. 'It was deafening and very frightening for a child. My job was to collect the large empty bobbins. We couldn't talk to one another, we were told what to do by sign language or by lip reading, which we all had to learn pretty quickly.'

As Mrs Williams was telling me this, I was reminded of the hospital consultant who had moved up from the south of England. One day, talking to colleagues in a confidential way, away from the patient's bedside, at what he thought was a discrete distance so the patient could not hear, he debated her possible treatment. Having finished his discussion he walked to the bed and before he could say anything, the patient said, 'it's bad news then, so what are you going to do about it.' He was non-plussed and his colleagues chuckled saying 'you always have to check whether your patients have worked in the textile mills first, they can lip read incredibly well at amazing distances.'

Mrs Williams was an intelligent lady, who clearly felt it deeply, that she had to leave school at a young age and thus was deprived of the one chance to, 'move up in the world.' She would have liked to have been a teacher but the nearest she got to this was her involvement with the Sunday school at her church which was a thriving community with over a hundred children attending. 'The great times were preparing all the children for the annual Whit Walks. All the churches would gather in procession and walk through the city on Easter Monday, or if you were Catholic, on the following Friday. The children would be dressed up in their Sunday best, there would be colourful banners, carried proudly by the men of the congregations, each huge, heavy banner depicting the church they represented. There were bass bands playing and huge crowds lined the streets watching, enjoying the day. Sadly now, these Walks no longer take place as they did.' I would listen to Mrs Williams as she recounted her tales. She didn't realise it but her enthusiastic story telling was worth all the technical breathing exercises I could give against her painful broken ribs. 'Get your husband to bring in your shoes tomorrow, we are going to walk. 'Oh good, see you tomorrow,' she said as she shuffled up the bed, and I walked away.

Next day, helping Mrs Williams into her dressing gown, she said 'do you think I could sit in that chair and could you wheel me up the road?' I knew which chair she was referring to before I turned my head.

'Yes, let's go. Good girl' she said happily.

We took a trip to the bathroom and as I closed the door, I said, 'give me a shout when you are ready.' A few minutes later, Mrs Williams sang out and I wheeled her back.

'By gum that's better, that's made my day,' she said appreciatively.

The day before the examination results were due was the day Mrs Williams was to go home. 'Don't forget to let me know how you got on,' she said as I treated her for the last time.

'I'll be seeing you in out-patients next week, just look after yourself until then,' I called after her, as she was wheeled away. She waved her good arm to all her friends in the ward and my last glimpse of that stoic lady was the porter pushing her in the wheelchair, her fractured wrist in its plaster, being held up in some sort of farewell salute.

After lunch, walking back to the wards, Sylvia, caught me up. She was breathless having choked down her lunch and dashed to the bank to be back in time to treat her first ward patient. 'Hello, anything interesting this afternoon?' I asked.

'I'm on the medical wards with a pretty mixed list,' replied my friend. 'I have a chap who thinks he is Charles the Second.'

'Not really,' I said, looking to see if my friend was kidding.

'Yes he does and what's more he looks like him too. He has long dark shoulder length hair, parted in the middle and it is in ringlets, and,' she added, 'he wears a sort of frilly white shirt, with lace cuffs instead of pyjamas'

'What do the other men in the ward think about it all?' I asked.

'Not much, they are giving him a wide berth, in case it's catching!' We were both laughing now at the thought of this spectacle.

'You had better watch out, he might mistake you for Nell Gwynne.'

Tall and slim, Sylvia looked down at herself, 'he would have to be as blind as a bat as well as daft but I'll watch him anyway.'

We were approaching the stairs now where she would go her way and I mine. 'What's on your list this afternoon?' She asked.

'Just the usual, post op chests but there is Mr Riley,' I added. Sylvia looked at me questioningly. 'Apparently, in a moment of boredom he did himself a mischief which had to be repaired under a general anaesthetic and because he's a smoker, now has a rotten chest too.' We were standing at the doors of Sylvia's ward as I had just remembered my first patient would be at x-ray.

'What mischief did he do' asked Sylvia intrigued.

'Well, he tried to make a ball point pen disappear via his penis and he was successful, unfortunately for him he couldn't retrieve it, he was in the bath' I added as if that explained the bizarre behaviour, plumping out the story. Sylvia's long legs sagged as she supported herself, leaning on the wall. 'Dear God,' she gurgled as I left her choking, crumpled against the radiator, her knees gone, helpless with laughter as tears streamed down her face. Obviously, Nell Gwynne, was in no fit state to treat Charles the Second.

CHAPTER FOURTEEN

Lucky Four

The day of the examinations results arrived and it required considerable will-power to get up and face the day knowing I would have to leave the house before the post arrived. Still there was no choice. With a dreadful dragging feeling I left the house to walk to the bus stop. Normally, I enjoyed the bus trip into the city centre. It was pleasant just to sit and gradually wake up, gently coming to terms with the dawning day.

I don't remember the journey that morning. Somehow I walked down Bridge Street, along Chapel Street, passed the policeman on point duty and only came to as I approached the door of the common room.

Several of our set had arrived already and were getting changed. 'Hello' I had said as I had walked into the room, only to be given a somewhat muted reply. A distant silence seemed to follow. I must have failed and they don't want to say anything I thought glumly to myself. I opened my locker and took out a clean white coat, it was one of a pile of six, so stiff with starch we had to shake it out and put our hands down the sleeves to prise them apart. As starched as they were, we liked them that way they stayed clean and neat looking much longer than the more limp but comfortable coats. I sat down, the coat across my knees and began to put the buttons in, forcing the metal button backs, through the starch filled islets. These metal button backs, played havoc with any decent underwear, snagging our silky slips, which we wore underneath.

Head down, totally engrossed in my own thoughts, the door was thrown open with a crash and the comforting size of Barbara appeared closely followed by Sylvia and Paula. As they flung themselves into the room they, were followed by Fiona. Congratulations, Barbara had called to me as she went to her seat in the corner. I gazed first at Barbara then at Fiona who sat down by my side, smiling. Suddenly, the room was full of noise. Everywhere people were arriving, throwing down their bags, shouting across the room. In the crush Barbara was struggling out of her over coat, her substantial chest straining against her bright blue jumper as she tried to wriggle her arms free in the confined space.

Galvanised by the hullabaloo, I called to her, 'do you mean I have passed?' There was a momentary lull in the thronging Babel, as everyone turned to look at me. 'Didn't you know three or four voices seemed to shriek at me?' I shook my head, 'I have to leave before the post arrives,' I explained. 'How has everyone else done?' Immediately the noise started up again, apparently only four of us had passed outright. Everyone had passed all but one subject, with the exception of one girl who had failed completely. No wonder there was a deathly hush when I first arrived I thought.

Needless to say, Fiona was among the successful and we sat there together quietly, letting the din flow over us, thankful we were among the lucky few.

There was an obvious bonding amongst those who had not been so lucky, and this sisterhood-in-adversity factor helped cheer them up. This kind of dissipation of disappointment was they hoped, shared by Bo. It was generally agreed that her inevitable wrath and sarcasm was not something to look forward to. In marked contrast to the common room din, we trooped across the quad in silence, our books clutched firmly about us, like a shield against the inevitable onslaught.

We trooped into the lecture and sat down to wait. Within seconds, the door opened and there was Bo in full, pristine white starched, regalia. Good morning, she winced. Her dark brown eyes taking in the scene, her eyebrows moving up and down constantly, while her lips formed the tight prune she adopted at times like this.

Without wasting any time she opened with, 'to those who have been successful, well done, the others I will see one at a time in my office later.' It had not occurred to us that the rest of the school had been taking exams and Bo would have more things to do than go into a public post mortem, there and then, with mere second year students.

The tension in the room lessened marginally when Bo, without any relaxation in her face, surprised us by launching into a short, forceful lecture on *kypho scoliosis* and its treatment. 'To diagnose the extent of the curvature of the spine, the patient must of course be stripped to the waist. Then standing in front and facing the long mirror, the patient should bend forward. The physiotherapist will get an accurate picture of the extent of spinal curvature, by looking at the patient's back in the mirror.' It sounded a bit unreal, almost with a hint of black magic but abruptly Bo finished the brief lecture by telling us, 'to go to the medical gym and check each other's back using this technique.' The results were interesting. It is surprising how many do have some degree of curvature of the spine. Mostly, though, we thought it was a plan of Bo's to divert us from exam mania. If so, it was effective.

For those of us who had been successful, the day passed pleasantly with both staff and patients congratulating us. I could hardly wait to get home. I knew my parents would be anxiously awaiting the results. Of course everyone was delighted when they heard the news and there were lots of hugs, smiles and 'I told you so's.' Most of all, I was personally very relieved. 'I had given it a try,' as my father had requested and now it was as obvious to me, as it had been to my parents, I was very happy in my chosen profession.

The passing of exams was only the hurdle, the race had to finish, so in no time at all, we were caught up in the never ending pace and order of hospital life. Now more than half our time was devoted to clinical treatment of patients. The spadework of anatomy was completed. It was easier now, as we treated our patients, we were applying the knowledge we had swotted over and this applied to pathology as well. It was easier to remember textbook conditions once you had treated a patient with the same. I found that I built up a mental library, which I could refer to, whether it was a baby critically ill with whooping cough or a first division footballer with torn cruciate ligaments. I found when meeting ex patients, even years later, I could remember their injury but not their name. And forgetting the old 'chestnut,' I didn't recognise you out of bed, I would ask 'how is it.' Invariably, the patient would touch their back or arm or whatever, telling me things were fine, giving me an instant picture of their old trauma. I was also learning the unwritten art of the bedside manner. I was learning the degree of injury and what you could realistically expect from the patient eventually. The winning of trust and cooperation was essential. It is not easy to explain to a paraplegic, who has been very active that there is a future in a wheel chair. I learnt you had to look at the hoped for end result of treatment in order to make an effective start. Of course most patients made a full recovery but for some, the physio had to start from where the patient was and not where they wanted to be.

CHAPTER FIFTEEN

Mistaken Identity

One morning, I was given a new patient to treat, he had been admitted overnight, and was called Zac. He was one of the West Indians who had come to this country to make a better life for himself. Although Zac was lying in bed, I could see he was a tall young man well over six foot. His milk-chocolate-coloured frame was smooth and muscular and his hair was cut neatly round his head.

There he was, lying quite flat on an inclined bed, head down, his neck totally immobilised. The foot of his bed was raised up on wooden blocks and to prevent him sliding down towards the wall, his legs were well secured with broad strips of sticking plaster stuck over long tapes. These tapes, in turn, were passed over pulleys and ended being fixed to heavy weights hanging down over the elevated foot of the bed. Thus poor Zac was tied to the bed, his body weight trying to slip down one end, while the heavy weights at the other made sure he didn't. There he was quite immobile, his large brown eyes and dark curly hair in sharp contrast to the snowy white pillow.

'Hello, I'm your physio,' I said, introducing myself.

'Hello,' he replied in a gentle voice, his handsome face seeming to split open with his wide smile, showing a magnificent set of white teeth. He licked his dry lips with a surprisingly pale pink tongue and I picked up his beaker.

'Like a drink?' I asked.

'Yes please, I've been waiting for someone to come along,' he replied gratefully. I steadied his beaker and fixed the concertina straw so Zac could take his long thirsty drink, no easy matter when you are lying down hill.

'What happened to you?' I asked as I put the beaker down on his locker.

He sighed and his large brown eyes rolled. 'We were playing cards at a friend's house last night, when a stranger burst in. I had my back to the door and I turned round to see what the noise was about when this man stabbed me in the back of my neck.' Zac blinked solemnly, 'mistaken identity, he thought I was someone else, a guy who owed him money.' He closed his eyes sorrowfully then opened them again to gaze at his feet. He related his story as if it was an every Wednesday night occurrence. I listened, without interrupting, as he told of the awful tragedy, I was pretty certain he didn't realise the seriousness of his injury or its implications. He knew he had been stabbed but as he was not sore, he thought it would only be a matter of days before he was up and about. 'I can't feel much in my lower half but then my legs have gone to sleep being tied to the bed.' He didn't mention he couldn't move his arms either. The only good news I thought to myself was my patient could at least breath by himself, but other than that, in light of the day after the night before, he looked like a classic quadriplegia, paralysed from the neck down and of course doubly incontinent. What rotten luck.

In the first few days nobody could predict with any accuracy what the final outcome of such an injury would be. There was swelling around the neck, which persisted for a few days, and it was hoped that when it subsided the pressure on the spinal cord, would be less and, if it hadn't been cut through, the degree of paralysis might not be absolute. The days passed and there was no improvement. Meanwhile it was my job to put his entire arm and leg joints through as full a range of movement as possible without disturbing his neck, to prevent his joints seizing up. Zac also had to be turned regularly to prevent bedsores, which required the most skilful nursing. Time was passing; still Zac had not been told he was a quadriplegia, probably, permanently. It made treating him doubly difficult.

Zac had not only lost all movement in his arms and legs but he also had lost all sense of feeling. He had lost sensation of pressure as well as heat and pain and consequently if he was subject to any injury, even a slight cut or scratch, without anyone being aware of it, could quickly cause infection.

Almost a week had passed and normally any paraplegia, quadriplegia or worse, tetraplegia, the inability to move their head or breath unaided, would have been transferred to a specialist unit. We were a teaching hospital with a specialist orthopaedic unit but not a hospital specialising in severe traumatic paralysis like Stoke Mandeville. The delay as far as Zac was concerned seemed to hinge on the possibility that he might be flown home to be with his family in Barbados.

Treating Zac was becoming more difficult as he became more depressed. Being a student, I was not allowed to say anything about his prognosis and trying to sound upbeat was becoming hollow. Patients do need to trust you to be honest with them in order to make any progress. Zac, became sullen and would not speak when spoken to and moved the only part of himself he could, turning his head to the wall. There, he would fix his eyes with a rigid middle distance stare. No amount of encouragement helped, he was slipping down a deep dark tunnel from which it was increasingly difficult to recall him. I totally sympathised with Zac, he was realising he would never walk again yet nobody had admitted this to him. To know from now on you can't feed yourself, scratch your nose, clean yourself after a bedpan or even read or write your own private letters is the most terrifying realisation. For Zac too, there was no nearby family to lend support and give comfort. Understandably, he did not want seemingly false jollity. It was only after Zac refused to eat, which after all was the only voluntary protest he could make, was the medical team forced into an explanation to talk about his future.

The next day or so were of black despair for Zac and yet I knew instinctively that now that he had been told exactly what the outlook was for him we could move on. The blackness lifted bit by bit. We could be honest with one another discussing the aims of treatment. Gradually through trust and honesty his confidence in me began to grow and gradually a friendship developed. The aims of treatment were to find out just what muscle power he had left and to develop it as much as possible. Any 'trick movements' which we frowned upon in the able bodied were now sought, encouraged and developed. Gradually Zac began to sit up propped up on special pillows and he began to take an interest in the ward about him. He graduated to standing in callipers, which would save his knees from buckling under him or worse from going into tight flexor spasms. It took three of us just to get his gear on and to get him upright. Time and again we were asked if it was worth all the time and effort especially as he couldn't support himself once he was standing, because of his paralysed arms. It was debatable, but just getting a disabled person upright to be able to see and speak to others on even terms, is in itself a tremendous step forward for a disabled person.

After three months of intensive physio, arrangements were made for Zac to return home to Barbados. He was visibly excited as I approached his bed and he couldn't wait to tell me he was going home. 'I'll be near my folks,' he said happily and I was glad for him. I sat down on the foot of his locker, as I usually did, to talk face to face and jokingly asked him if I could come too and he laughed his old cheerful laugh. As I listened to him, I quietly wondered how he would fare once he was home and I just hoped it would be as good as he thought it would be, and that the local hospital was good too because it would need to be. I had spent a great deal of time perched on the foot of his locker in the last few months. Whenever I had a few moments to spare and I was working on the wards, I would pop in to see Zac. I would read his letters to him or I would write those he dictated to me. Perched on his footlocker we were level and he could speak privately about his worries, tell me about his life 'back home,' and his hopes for the future, while I gave him snippets of news from the outside world. I fervently hoped that this young man, not much more than a youth, would find the joy and hope which he was so desperately seeking.

The day came when he had to fly home. As always I was sad to see the last of a patient that I had spent so many hours treating but I was pleased for him. He had tried his best with great fortitude and patience and richly deserved the national health flight home. As the porter and his accompanying nurse lifted him into his wheel chair, I joked about the unlikely possibility of me having a holiday in Barbados one day. His wide grin spread across his face, his wonderful teeth gleaming and he said 'I was to remember that I would always be welcome back at his home.' With that he was wheeled away.

Years later when I was working in a specialised unit, I discovered a very different approach, a mixture of warm sympathy and a realistic business like regime. Unlike Zac, the patients here were told from the beginning what the future held and in the very unlikely event we were proved wrong, great, what a bonus! From that moment the drive was on by all members of the team to gain as much as possible from the patient so that they would have as great independence in the outside world as humanly possible.

To optimise their independence, their nearest and dearest had to be members of the team too because a disabled person returning home will be joining what is then a disabled family and it will a hard slog for all. Of course the greatest hurdle the paraplegia or the blind will have to overcome will be us, the great British public, as any young mum pushing a baby buggy can confirm. There will be high steps and difficult doors in the shops, cars and dustbins left on pavements just to name a few obstacles which are no problem to the able-bodied but just try it in a wheel chair or with your eyes closed.

CHAPTER SIXTEEN

Rot Sets In

We were nearing the end of our second year when the first of our friends became engaged. It was Sylvia who started the rot, closely followed by Pauline. To be fair both of these girls had been going steady with their boyfriends long before coming to Salford. When they had left home to study, they had as Sylvia put it, 'had an agreement.'

There she was, the quietly pleasant, friendly girl from South Shields, grinning cheerfully. Her hair was close cropped almost like a boy's, the dark colour framing her pale freckled face. Sheila, who was sitting among us, was perched on the end of her seat with arm outstretched. At our request, she had extended her fingers to display her new engagement ring. 'No nothing had definitely been decided regarding the wedding day but of course it wouldn't be until after I've done my finals and gone home to work,' she informed us.

We were all wearing our gym kit. Sylvia's shorts were much shorter than any of the other girls and only emphasised the length of her long willowy legs. Sylvia was five foot seven in height and her legs seemed long and languid, the sort of limbs that models have and rarely found in physios. Since we first met, I had wondered how she had spent her childhood to end up with elegant limbs like that. She certainly had not indulged in athletics like me. True I had long legs but thanks to my passion for sprinting, my legs could hardly be described as languid by anyone, neither were her legs like Clare's, she, who had been a keen ice skater, nor like Fiona's the great horse woman amongst us.

I found being a physio teaches you to be like that. I constantly found myself weighing up people physically, first my fellow students of course but soon absolutely everyone. I found myself watching and analysing people, their build, their stance and how they walked, and why they walked and stood that way and I'm afraid I still do. One day I asked Sylvia about her fascinating legs and how she had spent her childhood. She chuckled, 'swimming,' she replied. Apparently, Sylvia, her boyfriend and the rest of their gang had spent every free moment, swimming. 'As we lived very near the sea, we never did anything else, the sea was everything to us, and I do miss it,' she added with a smile. I could imagine it too because her fiancé was a newly qualified marine architect, a profession not readily found in our student circles.

Looking back Sylvia was much more mature than the rest of us. Whenever the conversation lapsed into speculation about the opposite sex and in particular, 'the other,' usually amongst peals of laughter at the preposterousness of such an idea, Sylvia would be sitting with us, quietly smiling. We did not realise it then, but with the perfect vision of hindsight, she was not smiling with us, rather, at us. We were so incredibly green. Sylvia was a super person and how sad I felt when only few years later, I heard of her untimely death from cancer. She could only have been in her late twenties or early thirties.

A week or two later Paula became engaged to her policeman boyfriend. Paula was always the very picture of good health and vitality. She had brown curly hair, a bright rosy pink and white complexion and magnificent teeth. She had been going out with her boyfriend for ages and when she left Cumbria to study they had 'an understanding,' too. Paula stood, in the obligatory position; arm outstretched looking more radiantly healthy than usual, smiling away while we all dutifully admired her engagement ring.

Frankly, Fiona and I agreed, later when we were alone, they must be stark raving mad getting themselves tied down before they could discover what the big wide world holds for them.' We laughed heartily at Paula's smittence with the matrimonial state. 'I could no more bib and coo over every unsuspecting baby like she does, than fly to the moon,' my trusty friend said vehemently. I agreed, I thought of children as an, 'optional extra' in marriage, anyhow. We would watch Paula go into a sort of trance at the thought of marriage, babies and knitting woolly wellies. 'Ye Gods,' Fiona had whispered after one particularly drooling session, 'the girl's completely off her rocker.' I could only agree wholeheartedly.

Occasionally, Fiona and I would wonder about our femininity and apparent lack of maternal instinct, compared with Paula's that is, but the mood did not last long. Paula, going into one of her rapturous séances was enough to dispel any real doubts we might have had about us.

The rot was spreading. Three months later Clare became engaged. Clare was something of a loner. She was quiet, refined and had a shyness, that was often mistaken for aloofness. Within our set, she tended to migrate to our side. With Paula, Sylvia, Barbara, Fiona and I, Clare would join us to 'even things up,' particularly when we needed partners in practical sessions. Five foot three, with light brown hair, Clare was of trim build, she had blue eyes and an attractive light golden tan that never seemed to fade. Clare was always neat and tidy. Her shorts and shirt were never hastily bundled into her locker like ours were, but neatly folded and carefully placed. Our navy gear was lucky if it was washed once a term, Clare's shirts were a credit to Aertex and herself.

It seemed that recently, friends of Clare's family had come to visit along with their son. Clare and her parents had met the guests at the station and it was apparently, 'love at first sight,' for the young people. How lucky can you get, everyone knew and approved of everyone and all were delighted at the engagement and the thought of the forthcoming marriage. So there Clare was one morning in our corner of the common room, quietly displaying her large engagement ring at our request, giving us the briefest outline of how it had all come about. Why does everything run so smoothly for some people I wondered?

In a rare moment Clare had once told me that as a child she had developed tuberculosis. To aid her recovery she had been sent to school in the French Alps and it was there she had learned to skate and to speak her impeccable French. She had only mentioned to me about her having TB once and I kept her secret. It was clear from her manner, she had experienced all the social taboo and isolation which families had to endure when a member contacted the highly infectious 'consumption.'

In my last year at school, mass chest radiography was introduced to try to pick up any incidence of TB. It was still a huge scourge nationwide and two seemingly healthy boys in my class, alone, were found to be suffering from the early stages of the disease and had to go into a sanatorium. In at least two hospitals I have worked in, all members of the staff were offered mass radiography and at least one person in our department was found to have TB. Now because it is comparatively rare, mass x-ray is considered more of a health hazard than the disease itself but then, it was certainly instrumental in wiping out tuberculosis across the country.

Just before I started physiotherapy, my younger Brother, John, who was in his first year at a new school, somehow, suddenly contracted pneumonia. His pneumonia was quickly complicated by pleurisy, which in turn was not helped by an adverse reaction to the sulphonamide drugs, which he had been prescribed. It was the time before penicillin was readily available, it had been discovered of course but all supplies were being used by the armed forces, apparently.

My twelve-year-old Brother, John, was very ill and the doctor was coming twice a day. Gradually he improved and when he was up and about, he was sent to the Chest Clinic to have an x-ray to make sure no damage had been done to his lungs as the result of being so ill. There was damage. As a direct result of the pleurisy, he had a patch on his lung. I can remember the consultant holding up the x-ray, pointing out 'the shadow,' to my mother. The whole x-ray looked equally shadowy to me. We just sat there and listened as he announced that my brave brother would have to go away to another hospital, a sanatorium, for at least a year. Our world seemed to collapse about our ears. TB or consumption as it was commonly called, because it literally consumed the patient, was a highly infectious killer, and my twelve year old, brother had to be isolated.

I was very close to John and felt deeply for him. He was going to be sent away to a sanatorium in Abergele, some seventy miles away. There was no choice, for what was a vital year away from home and school. The consultant went on to tell us he would spend the first six months on complete bed rest, no getting up for any reason including the toilet and if all goes well John will be allowed up gradually during the next six months.

We had one bit of good luck when our GP managed to find a small sanatorium just for children where we were allowed to visit once a week on Saturdays. This sanatorium had just opened in the countryside about twenty miles from where we lived, which was less frightening for children than the huge sanatoria for adults and was of great help to us because it was so much nearer to our home.

John along with other children, spent all day outside, in the fresh air, the beds arranged in a row under a long veranda. They were never brought into the ward. Hail, rain or snow that's where they ate, slept, did their school work and, in the case of John's best friend, in the next bed, died.

The food at the hospital was especially nutritious to try to prevent the TB progressing. It was an indicator you were getting no worse if you were able to maintain your weight and if you were actually putting on weight, the signs were you were actually beating the consumption. During the second six months, John seemed to be practically force fed. He changed from being the skinny, leggy twelve-year-old, as we all had been at the same age, to a veritable Billy Bunter. When my parents queried his weight gain, they were assured it was an encouraging sign and were told that when a patient puts on weight he is winning the fight. For John though, it proved to be a lasting nightmare, he struggled with a weight problem thereafter.

All through the year, week in week out, we trekked to the 'hospital,' my mother forbidding us to use the term 'sanatorium,' 'because we would be treated like lepers.' Kindly friends would enquire after John from time to time and we dutifully told them he was recovering well from his pneumonia. Occasionally some clever adult would take me to one side and in a confidential manner try to question me further. However their ploy was to no avail, we had all been well primed by my mother as to what to say. Up until then I thought my mother had exaggerated the problem and that she was a product of a bygone age regarding other people's attitudes but we soon found out about the stigma the hard way.

For what seemed like years afterwards the whole family had to have chest x-rays every six months to make sure none of us had contracted the disease. It was explaining my absence to Clare, from the hospital one morning, when I had been for my check-up that had precipitated her confiding in me. Yes, I could certainly understand Clare's reticence in talking about her past medical history. Of course nowadays patients are just treated with antibiotics and unless they are very ill when diagnosed, can go about their daily lives more or less.

How things have changed.

CHAPTER SEVENTEEN

Social Rounds

Engagement rings and all other jewellery, for that matter, were strictly forbidden. Every morning our engaged friends went through a somewhat exaggerated ritual of taking off their rings and pinning them, with a huge safety pin, to the inside of their white coat pocket. If for some reason the coat had to be changed or we had to change into gym kit the performance was repeated. At the end of the day the ritual was reversed and judging from Paula's hypnotic state during this palaver it was a dress rehearsal for the marriage ceremony.

Fiona and I were not idle on the boyfriend front, it was just that we had not found anyone we could remotely consider spending our lives with.

I was busy in what spare time I had, being on the local YHA executive and also helping inner city children with reading at the University settlement. On Saturday nights I would often go to the university hops and Jane, my friend from school days, now doing teacher training, would join me when she was home for the weekend. That was until Jane's mother began to think I was a bad influence on her. This was awful, as our parents had been friends for years, and 'things' were getting tense. 'Quite unjustifiably,' as I later explained to my parents and so it transpired.

Jane, in her own words, was no raving beauty, with brown hair and glasses. She was a girl ahead of her time, never bothering to buy a bra because she considered her bosom too inadequate to necessitate throwing good money away on such. The result was not exactly devastating but rather of the straight up and down look of the nineteen twenties. When we were having one of our confidential chats she would, on rare occasions, say hold on while I clean my specs, assuring me that when her glasses were not on her nose, not only could she not see anything but she couldn't hear too well either. For all that, Jane had a lively personality and we got on well together.

One evening, when we were together at a dance, Jane met an Indian graduate. They fell in love and went out together for weeks. Some months later the graduate suddenly took himself off to work in Germany for six months, and Jane never heard from him until he was about to come back when he wrote to my bereft friend asking her to marry him. Happy, she agreed. He returned to Manchester, as promised, only to disappear to India a couple of weeks later without any explanation what-so-ever and never, it seems, to be heard of again. Jane was heartbroken and her mother angry at treatment of her daughter and therefore me. Secretly, I believe, her mother was very relieved at the outcome. Bit by bit, Jane's mother realised I was not to blame and said as much to me and to my parents, who reassured her they had understood her worry.

A couple of years later, Jane came to visit me, when I had qualified and was working in Berkshire. Clearly she was in love. She had met a newly graduated architect from Yorkshire and everything was perfect. Later we all met up at their wedding. They were married, in sunny Manchester, later to live happily ever after in North Yorkshire. And once more Jane's mother looked on me with grace and favour.

As for Fiona, she had met James at a hunt ball. She assured me that 'he had all the sexual charm of a string bean, six foot three and he drooped in the middle.' I couldn't help laugh with her, as she went on to say 'his floppy hair sags into his eyes and he has a large Adam's apple that goes up and down like a lift with a half broken cable, as he talks.'

'What is it exactly, that is endearing you to James?' I had asked, trying to look earnest and understanding.

She took a deep breath. 'Well he comes from a good family' She said thoughtfully, 'and did go to Oundle, you know. Besides, he will do for the time being!' She added pragmatically.

'Why what's coming up?' I asked.

'Another hunt ball and,' she continued, 'at least he can be guaranteed not to shovel his peas with his fork!' She finished seriously.

I nodded and smiled at the same time, good old Fiona and to look at her butter wouldn't melt in her mouth.

CHAPTER EIGHTEEN

Professional Footballers et al

It was the Ball season and I had been invited to my first formal, action was needed fast. During our lunch hour a couple of days later, Fiona and I made a dash to Saint Ann's Square in the centre of Manchester. I had seen a blue ball gown that had taken my fancy, beautiful blue organdie with shimmering silver threads running through the lovely floaty material. To be able to afford this masterpiece of haute couture, I had cashed some carefully hoarded saving certificates. I had given the matter a great deal of thought and there just was no alternative, I had to break into my emergency fund.

I had been invited to the 'formal' by some one I had recently met at the university. He was very pleasant, tall, and a somewhat precise graduate. In fact when I first met him at the local hop it was clear he wasn't a student but had been. When I asked him, 'when did you graduate,' he rattled off three dates in quick succession ending that he had taken his PhD when he was twenty-three. He went on to say 'he should have been awarded it when he was twenty-two but they made him wait'. He was also a great ballroom dancer and very keen on 'formals.' To go to this function meant breaking the bank and break the bank it did. Still you only live once I decided.

Missing our lunch, we hurried into town and made our way to St Ann's Square. Collecting ourselves at the doorway we entered the shop and I asked to see the gown of my choice. 'Certainly madam,' came a somewhat aloof response and Fiona and I looked at one another as we were shown into a desperately small changing room.

A moment or two later, the shop assistant appeared with the blue creation and mercifully left us to it. I struggled out of my outdoor clothes and then my jumper and skirt and handed everything to Fiona. Somehow or other I managed to get the dress over my head, pulling and smoothing the layers down. I stood there trying to do up the zip, at the same time trying to assess the overall effect.

'Why didn't you bring a strapless bra?' the squashed, inert Fiona had asked caustically as she stared at the apparition in the facing mirror. 'Especially when trying on a strapless gown.'

'Hmm,' I muttered glumly, my white bra straps were detracting from the overall picture of what I had hoped it to be, one of glamour and allure. I didn't like to confess to Fiona I did not possess such an item of underwear but that it was definitely next on my shopping list.

'Well are you going to take it or not?' Asked Fiona briskly. 'Time's running out!'

I stood there trying to drape the stole, which went with the evening dress, round my shoulders, muttering to myself why such an expensive gown should have such a skimpy stole. It beats me, penny pinching lot.

'Yes' I said, scrambling back into my clothes, which Fiona was handing me item by item. We eventually emerged from the suffocating cubbyhole, which passed for a changing room, hot and pink. Paying for the dress, I asked the assistant to keep the enormous box for me promising to collect it later that afternoon.

'Quick we have less than ten minutes to get back!' said Fiona. We galloped out of St Ann's Square, and as we turned onto Deansgate we saw a green Salford bus coming our way.

'Quick, stick a paw out or it will go by!' I gasped. I was still trying to retrieve my coat belt, which would not come to heel. We clambered aboard the bus and flopped down on the nearest seats. I glanced at my watch and said 'we should be all right for time' Fiona nodded in agreement.

Already we were moving down Bridge Street and, a moment or two later, we were at the hospital. Hurtling up the front steps through the front door, unbuttoning our coats as we hurried down the corridor. There was not a moment to lose, into our shirts, shorts and pumps, retracing our steps down the corridor, turning towards the courtyard at the rear of the hospital. Out of the building, we dashed down the cobbled street. Although it was cold outside, we didn't notice it. I often wondered what the people thought who lived in the terraced houses, about our mad dashes down to the Adelphi Lads' Club, so sparsely dressed even in the bleakest weather.

We pushed open the heavy doors of the Lads' Club, and were immediately met by the characteristic smell of the large dusty spacious building. I never discovered where all the other doors lead to that confronted us as we entered this immense place but there certainly wasn't time to find out now. Up the concrete flight of stairs we leapt, two at a time and banged open the large heavy doors of the gym.

The male students were waiting for us, standing in the corner of the vast space. They had been there throughout the lunch break playing indoor football. One of the students, a charming man with total alopecia, was hanging upside down on the wall bars, his improbable ginger wig askew. This hairpiece was fascinating, firstly the shade was like no colour that I had ever seen and secondly it seemed to defy gravity, clinging with an unknown force miraculously, to his noble, high gloss, hair free cranium.

Mrs McGinty, our lecturer in physical education, was also there talking to two or three of the male students. She was probably about fifty, medium height, skinny, with a sort of fair, greying hair, which she wore in a loose bun at the nape of her neck. As usual she was wearing her short grey gym skirt, a grey aertex top and on her feet, grey light canvas slip-ons which were secured across the instep by a broad band of elastic. Around her neck she carried a referee's whistle, which hung across her not quite supported bosom, like a badge of office.

Mrs McGinty blew her whistle and called us to gather round. If we female students had been on our own she would have settled down to making a veritable meal of her speech only interrupting the incredibly boring monologue with her loose chesty smokers cough. We would sit there hypnotised, staring at her feet as she paused at every other word to let the significance of what she was saying sink in. She emphasised every syllable with a circling action of her ankles, first one foot then the other, our eyes locked on to this exaggerated movement. Altogether we must have spent days, if not weeks, mesmerised by her feet being circled through their full range of movement, ending her endless speeches with full flexion and dorsiflexion of each foot in turn. At each lecture to her female students, we could be quite certain that both feet had the full treatment during the soporific drone. But not today, 'the gods be praised,' the male students, most of whom were considerably older than us, wouldn't stand for it. During mixed lectures or gym sessions, Mrs Mcginty would always address herself to the men. We were just extras on set.

For all that, Mrs McGinty was an excellent gymnast and, in the practicalities, no mean teacher. Because it was a mixed session, we soon had the volley ball net slung across the gym and for the next hour we would have a frantic game with Mrs McGinty darting about, blowing her whistle and generally keeping a tight grip on the proceedings. In volleyball we were equal to the men. Any game that involved feet and kicking the heavy leather football, the men ran rings round us but then they would. Some of them were professional footballers after all. Finally Mrs McGinty blew her whistle for the end of the afternoon session. Everything was packed away, the great edifice was locked up and off we went. We walked back to the hospital, down the cobbled Salford streets, glowing pink, hot and unbelievably healthy in the fading light of a winters late afternoon.

As soon as we had changed, for the last time, back into our *civvies*, Fiona and I hurried out on our respective ways, she to get the bus to the railway station and I to get the bus back to the centre of Manchester. I usually walked from Salford, to save bus fares but today I was on a mission, first to collect my beautiful ball gown.

Clutching the huge cardboard box containing the exquisite creation, I hurried from St Ann's square and headed up Market Street to Lewis's department store. I dashed up the escalator to the first floor to 'soft furnishings, dress patterns and materials.' As I stepped off the escalator, I made a bee-line to where I could see the bales of materials arranged in colourful rows along the back wall. Keeping my fingers crossed I hurried over to the rolls of glorious silks and organdies, hoping I would find the exact shade of blue I was looking for. I was in luck. Sure enough as I removed the tissue paper from the corner inside my dress box I could see the exact colour peeping out. The material on the bale was forty eight inches wide, just right. I ordered four yards, deciding that if I was going to have a stole at all, the effect might as well be elegant as well as dramatic.

Feeling very pleased with myself, I hurried away up to the next floor, lingerie. I asked the assistant for a selection of strapless bras in my size. The woman returned moments later with an armful for me to choose from. The styles ranged from padded, satin armour plating to a wisp of totally unsupported lace and silk. The latter was very pretty but clearly so hazardous that I chickened out and chose three more realistic garments to try on. I elected to buy a pretty but smooth bra that would show no lines under my silky dress. What is more the bra stayed with me when I breathed in and out, lifted up my arms and best of all, when I spun round, it did not stay facing due south. Well one never knows, I thought as I gave myself a final look, imagine jiving, I was not ready for that sort of mortification.

Tired but very pleased with my purchases, I walked across Piccadilly to catch the bus home. As I found a seat, I clutched my precious parcels about me, content in my work and happy in my shopping. Life seemed very good.

CHAPTER NINETEEN

May Ball

My parents were just about to leave the house to have dinner with friends when Roland arrived. He was the bright PhD that had invited me to the University Ball and to which end I had blown my savings on the now famous blue evening gown.

Simultaneously as he arrived on the doorstep, they had opened the front door. I who had been waiting and watching for him at my bedroom window, saw him arrive and shot downstairs to open the door. They stood there in amazement as the long streak of blue hurtled down the stairs to open the door but my parents had beaten me to it. I don't know who was the more startled, my parents finding a stranger on the doorstep or Roland who had his hand poised to ring the doorbell.

Of course in the last few days I had mentioned I was going to go to a ball with someone new but it obviously had not registered. Well there he was, tall, elegant in his evening suit, equally surprised. Roland stood there clutching a small cellophane box of delightful fresh flowers. Roland continued to stand there not quite sure whether he had the correct house.

'Er you had better come in young man,' my father said, collecting himself. My father always addressed my escorts as *young man*, he could never remember their names and had long since given up trying. I had resigned myself to all my male friends being so addressed, it had embarrassed me initially when he had forgotten my boy friends names but I was more embarrassed when he addressed them by someone else's name. So my father played it safe. Anyhow this form of address sorted the men from the boys, I decided. The keen and courteous stayed the course recognising in my father his old fashioned charm. The flippant and casual, that might have taken umbrage, quickly disappeared and were no loss at all.

I showed Roland into the living room catching my mother's smile of approval as she closed the front door behind her. Roland stood there and gravely presented me with the lovely corsage, which he had so thoughtfully brought me. I was very impressed, the flowers were delightful and had obviously been chosen with great care.

I went back upstairs to collect my evening bag and gloves. I carefully pinned the flowers into place then draping my luxuriant stole across my shoulders gave myself a twirl and final glance in the mirror. Thankfully, I found the reflection reassuring.

'You look wonderful,' said Roland quietly as he came to meet me as I entered the room. He took hold of both my hands and I found myself smiling with pleasure and thinking that there is everything to be said for gallantry.

I enjoyed the evening enormously. Roland was an excellent dancer and as soon as the orchestra started he would lead me to the dance floor and sweep me along across the room. Not for him waiting until the floor filled up to shuffle anonymously in a crowd. Roland told me on our second date he had concentrated so much on his education and getting a PhD as soon as possible, that he forfeited a great deal by way of a social life. He was only too aware that he was a specialist in his field but needed to broaden his horizons so he had taken up ballroom dancing. Characteristically, he applied himself, single-mindedly to his new past time, and was a gold medallist when we had met. So there I was at my first ball, being taken a firm hold of and swept across the empty dance floor as soon as the music started, leaving the close encounters of the smooch kind until later in the evening when there wasn't room to do anything else.

Roland was a very individual person, in some ways a product of too early specialisation when he was at school. He had won a place at university when he was very young only to find they would not take him until he was a year older. That September found him back at school, disconsolate. Suddenly the powers-that-be had a change of heart and by October a month later he had enrolled at the University. In the minimum time possible he gained a BSc, MSc and then his PhD, the authorities making him wait before he was awarded his doctorate because of his age.

About his academic brilliance there could be no doubt but as my knowledge of pure chemistry was severely limited, I felt that there was some lack of spontaneous conversation. I soon realised Roland was incapable of socialising as I had been brought up to but then I had been to boarding school where you socialised to survive.

To be fair Roland recognised all this hence his ballroom dancing skill. He was now turning his attention to classical music, which, as I belonged to a musical family, was great news. For him, it was impossible just to get a smattering of a subject so he could chat to people, that was just being flippant and superficial. A subject or pastime had to be to be thoroughly researched, weighed and finally exhausted. It was not a conscious thing for him, it was just part of his make-up.

I suppose even at that early stage in our relationship, I knew he was not the man for me ultimately. Meanwhile I had a wonderful time at the ball, dancing the night away until the last waltz. Being the sort of person that usually fell apart if I did not get to bed by midnight, I could not believe it was two o'clock in the morning and time to go.

We walked from the great hall across the quadrangle to where his car was parked. What a memorable night it had been. It had been my first real ball and with a thoughtful companion who was a marvellous dancer. My ball gown, which judging from the admiring glances I had received, was a great success. So much for the white-bra-strap apparition that Fiona had first commented on.

As we drove home, I began to wonder if Roland had enjoyed the evening as much as I had and whether he would ask me out again. I began to hope he would, although I knew he was not a kindred spirit, a feeling that is so difficult to describe yet so recognisable when you discover it.

The car drew to a stop outside my home. He switched off the engine and turned to me. Being a bit nervous I did not wait for him to speak but just thanked him for a lovely evening.

'I'm so glad you enjoyed it, because I did, very much indeed,' he said earnestly and paused for a minute. 'Would you like to come out for the day on Sunday?' He asked.

I was delighted on two counts, firstly, he wanted to take me out again which is always flattering and secondly my dancing couldn't have been all that bad either.

'Yes, I would love to,' I answered truthfully. He let himself out of the car and came round to my side and opened my door to help me out. We walked up to the porch, stopped and he kissed me.

'Good morning,' he said quietly, 'I'll call for you on Sunday.'

CHAPTER TWENTY

Morning After

Next morning I dragged myself off to the hospital feeling completely whacked. One thing was certain, there was never any slump in hospital business and I knew that ahead of me would be the usual strenuous day.

As I changed into my hospital gear, I mentally arranged in what order I would treat my patients. I would definitely not treat Mrs Wilkinson with a slipped lumbar disc first, because she was chronically depressed, and any one treating her for a long period of time, as I had been, was in danger of ending up the same way. Nor could I face Mr Bird, the recovering hernia. His hearty, rapid-fire-type repartee was just too much before nine o'clock today. That left the two head injuries, both deeply unconscious. Sadly but certainly, they were not in a position to engage me in scintillating conversation before the day was aired.

Liam then, was my first patient to be treated I decided. He was fifteen years old and fighting for his life. He had borrowed a friend's moped and, for a moment or two, wobbled and fallen under the wheels of a passing truck. He had been deeply unconscious for seven days, since being admitted. Liam was just beginning to surface again not obviously to an outsider perhaps, the degree was far too slight for that, but to us, there were faint but positive signs. He was responding to painful stimulus, the deepest of all reflexes, such as a slight pinprick and because of his youth the outlook allowed hope.

Liam was no longer on a life support machine, he was now breathing on his own, but he did need to have his lungs cleared. Anyone lying so inert collects secretions in their lungs, which in normal circumstances are coughed away so they have to be cleared for them. To prevent pneumonia developing at least or drowning in their own secretions at the very worst, a narrow tube is inserted down the bronchus and the phlegm cleared. Before I could do this though I had to make sure the air pockets in his lungs were as clear as possible. Greeting Liam as I entered the freezing room, I turned off the fan that was keeping my patient cool. So often with head injuries the part of the brain that regulates body temperature had been affected and Liam was burning up. He was lying there under a single sheet just to protect his modesty. His eyes were still somewhat swollen, the blue bruising beginning to turn yellowy brown. On his head he had a skullcap of thick cotton padding to protect the areas where the surgeon had relieved the pressure on the brain by drilling burr holes through his skull. Without this skilful intervention, Liam certainly would have died.

'Hello Liam how are you today' I asked as I gently turned him onto his side and taking his ribs between my hands gently vibrated his chest making him catch his breath and cough. 'There we are,' I said, as I literally gave Liam a breather. Doing this caused the sticky secretions to move towards the bronchus so that I could clear his chest with suction later. I went round to the other side of the bed and turned Liam over so his right side was uppermost and repeated the treatment talking to him all the while. It is the rule that you always talk to unconscious patients as if they can hear everything even if they cannot respond. It is well documented even deeply unconscious patients have heard bedside conversations and have said as much once they were able to speak.

Having finished the postural drainage, I turned Liam over so that he was again lying on his back. I switched on the suction machine and passing a rubber tube into his bronchus, cleared his chest of phlegm. This certainly isn't the most pleasant job in the world for the physiotherapist, especially first thing in the morning but it has to be done. The patient of course, being unconscious, is blissfully unaware of this unpleasant activity.

Now that Liam's chest was clear, my next job was to make sure his joints were kept mobile so when he regained consciousness and wanted to move his arms and legs he would be able to do so. Up until now there had been no response when I asked him to move but today as I took hold of his right hand his fingers flexed round my thumb, rather like a baby would do. Actually to say it was a movement was overstating it but his fingers definitely flickered in response to my request. 'Well done Liam try that again,' I urged and he did. Great, I thought, Liam is on his way back.

I arched my back and stretched up, it had taken a good half hour to treat Liam but what a result, slight as it was. I put the single sheet back over Liam, switched back on the cooling fan and then his little tape recorder playing his favourite tunes. His brother had brought it in at my suggestion just to try to trigger some responses.

'See you later Liam,' I said patting his shoulder, 'keep those fingers moving' and left.

Next on my list was Tommy Dale, the head injury in the other side ward. He had been admitted about eight weeks ago as the result of a horrendous traffic accident. Tommy was fifty-five years old and seemed to make a steady recovery in the first few days, gradually surfacing, so much so that after three weeks he was able to walk slowly about the ward. He had graduated from having two strong physios shoring him up, to him staggering around the ward on his own. True his gait resembled that of a zombie but he was progressing, eventually pushing the afternoon tea trolley while the orderly did the tea pouring. Suddenly one afternoon, while he was watching television in the day room with fellow patients, Tommy collapsed. He was taken back to his side ward where he had lapsed into deep unconsciousness within minutes. The doctors were called at once and he was given a lumbar puncture straight away. This showed the spinal fluid to be the colour of dirty washing up water instead of being the clear, pale fluid it should have been. Obviously Tommy was in big trouble.

The doctors tried everything but Tommy stayed deeply comatosed. If there was a change at all it was only a change for the worse. As the days passed Tommy began to flex up more and more in the prenatal position. The treatment was the same for Tommy as it had been for Liam. I had first to clear his chest then try to keep his arms and legs supple but Tommy was a lot heavier. Try as I might I was losing the battle. Tommy was beginning to curl up in the foetal position more and more. The nurses were turning Tommy regularly to prevent bedsores but he was losing weight so rapidly that his bones seemed to be poking through his skin and no amount of artificial feeding was putting meat on his skeletal body. I was keeping up my normal practise of greeting and speaking to my patient but it all seemed to no avail and poor Tommy was becoming more and more exhausting to treat. To try moving one hip for example set off a tremendous spasm in the other and I had to watch I didn't get hit with the opposite knee, which would flip up into my face if I wasn't ready for it. Added to his problems was the fact that now Tommy was doubly incontinent and involuntary spasms of his legs resulted in disaster. It was a full time job keeping him dry and clean. I left Tommy as comfortable as possible telling him I would soon be back. As I left I walked into his wife and daughter, I felt very sorry for them.

Tommy had been on the point of going home before his relapse. For his nearest and dearest, Tommy's set back was a second desperate trauma. His family could only look on as we tried everything we could for him. I spoke to them as I washed my hands; they had been outside waiting for me to finish treating Tommy. I had got to know them quite well over the last three or four weeks, and I just wished I could have given them some hopeful news when they asked how he was?

I left the ward and made my way down to the dining room for my coffee break. I sagged into a vacant chair near the door. David, one of the professional footballer students and as nice a chap as you could wish to meet, sat down and asked me what was up? I told him I had just been treating Tommy Dale. I did not have to say any more, David was on his feet asking me if I took sugar in my coffee? He was already on his way to the serving hatch for me. He returned with the steaming cup and placed it down in front of me.

'Get outside that!' He said in his gentle Lancashire accent. 'You'll soon feel better.' I smiled and gratefully thanked him.

Soon my friends began to come in for their coffee break but I had a heavy list so as soon as I had finished my coffee it was back to the wards.

Mrs Thomas was my next patient, a dear soul who looked forward to her treatment with a most flattering eagerness. I knew as I pushed open the ward doors she would be watching to see if it was I coming to give her treatment. As soon as she saw me her face would light up with pleasure in the most endearing way. Even if I was on my way to treat someone else there was always a cheery aside as I passed by. Physiotherapists' can look forward to a miserable pittance salary wise once they had finished their expensive studies but it is the Mrs Thomas's of this world that go a long way towards compensating for the inability to pay the rent.

Mrs Thomas had arthritis. 'Something shocking!' She had told me that on her first treatment. 'I was fifty,' she started, 'I suppose it was 'the change.' I nodded. 'I had five children,' she continued, 'well, six but one was a flower.' I must have looked blank at the word 'flower,' which was new to me. She leaned towards me and said confidentially, 'born dead, a lovely boy, a beautiful flower he was. We lived in a cottage in the country, it was four hundred years old. No running water just a pump near the front door and of course no gas or electricity. My husband worked hard when he could find work but it wasn't easy, now he has gone. I managed pretty well until my hips started playing up but in the last few months I have had to live with my daughter and her family, it's not the same you know.'

I had listened to Mrs Thomas without interrupting her, it was quite clear she was not complaining but in her own graphic way putting me in the picture. She had come into hospital for a hip replacement. Although Mrs Thomas was elderly, her still strong arms and clear complexion illustrated how hard she had worked all her life but I could see how fit it had kept her. On this particular morning I thought she looked a bit worried.

'What's the matter?' I asked. 'Is it the new exercises?'

'I've got a funny feeling in my metatarsals, a sort of prickly feeling.' She earnestly put it. It sounded like pressure on a nerve supply, not something to be ignored. Mrs Thomas had her hands tucked under her knees as she was gazing at her toes. I picked up first on foot then the other, there was a pressure mark across her ankles.

'It's alright,' I reassured her, 'you, must have been resting awkwardly in the night.' I gave her feet a vigorous rub while gently admonishing her for lying so still.

'My, that feels good.' She said as she lay back on her pillows with contentment written all over her face. 'A real treat.' She closed her eyes and seemed for a moment or two to be asleep then she gave a snort and opened her eyes. 'I'm so sorry.' She apologised. 'We had a noisy night last night with emergencies being brought in and it's the lights, I can't sleep with the lights on and I know the nurses must be able to see.'

'Don't worry,' I said, 'I quite understand, hospitals are not the most restful places.' It was the old problem, if you did manage to get to sleep you are woken to have temperatures and pulses taken or perhaps be given medication then to crown it all you are woken early to get things underway before the day staff come on duty at seven thirty. During the day there are the cleaners, the newspaper rounds, medicines, bed making, going to x-ray, and junior doctors' rounds before the consultant's round or even having physio treatment, then of course, visitors. No there is not a lot of rest in hospital. My sympathies were certainly with Mrs Thomas, there is nothing like a good night's sleep to make you feel better.

As Mrs Thomas was telling what a bad night everyone had the night before, I was reminded of a previous patient of mine. Herbert was a historian by profession and knew that all the great historical houses often claimed, as a matter of pride, rightly or wrongly, to have been visited by Queen Elizabeth the first. After a couple of particularly noisy and sleepless nights he decided to do something about it and make a gentle protest. He was being discharged that day so theoretically it did not matter any more, still he wanted to make his point. Herbert wrote out a large poster and stuck it on the wall above his head just before the consultant's ward round was due. In large bold print it said, 'Queen Elizabeth 1st, did not sleep here and neither did I.' The consultant laughed sympathetically and moved on.

Remembering my late night as I drew back the curtains round Mrs Thomas's bed, I agreed with Mrs Thomas's sentiments. I was pretty well shot myself, getting to bed in the early hours. What wouldn't I give to be curled up with a cosy hot water bottle in my snug bed at home right now? I looked at my watch, eleven forty, 'come on Mrs Thomas let's put your socks and shoes on and we will see if you can dance the light fantastic.'

'Right love' she chuckled and with that she gingerly let me help her swing her legs over the side of her bed. I put on her shoes, handed her, the crutches. She took a deep breath and off we went.

CHAPTER TWENTY-ONE

Kippers

As I arrived back in the department, I heard hoots of laughter coming from one corner. I saw Fiona amongst the group who were laughing as I strolled over and asked her what was going on? She told me 'somebody has sent Bo a box of Manx kippers from the Isle of Man. It has been delivered directly to her office so we think it must be from one of the men students but nobody is claiming the glory.'

'Yes it will be the male students four of them went to the Isle of Man for a short break last weekend. I don't know where they stayed but I wouldn't put it past them to send something as pungent as that to Bo', offered Barbara.

As if on cue, Bo's office door was flung open and there was our magnificent principal striding out holding a coarse wooden box at arm's length. She marched over to us noting, no doubt, that we were standing around apparently with nothing to do. We were in luck though, her face had a broad smile.

'Somebody has kindly sent me a box of kippers from the Isle of Man,' she said, clearly quite pleased that someone had thought about her enough to send her this gift. She put the box down and turned it over to show us. 'I wonder who it is from? There is no name of the sender on it other than the packers label,' she said. Trying to hide our amusement, we all peered at the smelly box. Sure enough there was only the dispatcher's note on the outside of the box which was well glued down and marked only with greasy fingerprints but it was clearly addressed to Miss Bodoano, The Principal of The Salford School of Physiotherapy.

After we had all examined the kippery box we assured her that we had no idea who the generous benefactor was but I agreed, perhaps too fervently, that it was a very kindly thought.

'Well,' said Bo beaming, 'I won't be able to get through all these myself perhaps you would like a pair each for your supper night.' Bo had addressed her query to Barbara, Sylvia and Paula whom she knew lived away from home.

Taken somewhat aback, they had automatically answered a thank you very much. 'Good, call at my office before you leave this afternoon and I will divide them out' Bo replied.

'I hope you know what you have let us in for, accepting those kippers?' Paula had said to Barbara accusingly as Bo walked off.

'Why, man, they are delicious!' retorted the girl from South Shields.

'I know that, you fool, but if we try to cook those in our room it isn't going to be a secret for long is it,' said the exasperated Paula.

'Man, she's right, they will be able to smell the kippers cooking all over the Y.W. and the smell will last for days,' said Sylvia in her gentle Geordie accent.

'We'll worry about that afterwards,' said Barbara not being put off the thought of a free tasty supper, then trying to placate her friends said 'I'll go and collect them from Bo, this afternoon if you like?'

We never did find out who the benefactor was but our friends assured us they did indeed taste wonderful even if Paula had to spend most of the evening whirling the tea towel round her head in an attempt to dispel the aroma, to prevent them being expelled from the hostel.

CHAPTER TWENTY-TWO

Physio To Teacher, It's Faster

The next major external examinations loomed. They took place just after the second year and like the first external examinations, they had to be passed in their entirety. These exams consisted of written papers on histology, pathology the study of disease, and the treatment of all or any medical conditions. Then there were also oral examinations or vivas, which were always an unknown quantity as it depended so much on the examiners personality and their method of verbal inquisition. Somehow, though, as worrying as the exams were, they did not seem to hold the same unholy terror as the first major hurdle had, at the end of the first year. It was no use bleating at home in any case, my family seemed to take it for granted I would sail through.

All the students who had failed part of the first exams a year ago had retaken them and were either successful or had left altogether, no quarter given. Those of us remaining were expected to be successful in our profession with a considerable degree of excellence. So, as we entered the third year, we were all on a par professionally speaking.

Never the less it had been a sad day some months earlier when Jane had to leave. Jane was sandy haired, of medium build with a quiet warm Lancashire accent. She was conscientious and got on well with her patients but somehow or other just could not pass her electrotherapy exam. In a way the failing of this exam was somewhat unfair, it was ninety per cent physics with a large electro mechanics component. Yes, it was obvious we needed to know the therapeutic effects of the various electrical treatments which we give to our patients and the types of electrical currents responsible for each of the medical conditions we were treating or about to treat remedially. Having said that, in practise we were not allowed to touch a faulty machine or even to change a plug. We always had to call the electrical department, it was all to do with insurance apparently.

The day Jane left was a miserable day for us all. She was such a nice person, if only she could have squeezed through. We all felt she would have made a good physio. Jane stood there looking the very picture of dejection, 'I'll end up teaching after all' she had said despondently. All her family had been or were teachers and Jane had wanted to break the mould. Apparently Bo had sent for her and had given her the bad news, which according to Bo, was that Jane was not cut out to be a physiotherapist. I felt particularly sympathetic to Jane remembering a somewhat similar interview with Bo three years ago and how I too had felt that the bottom had dropped out of my world. We all sat there trying to think of some words of comfort.

'Never mind, if you do go to college next term, you will be finished before us not to mention earning a salary sooner' I said desperately trying to cheer her up.

'I suppose so,' she nodded glumly. In those days, students at training college qualified in two years whereas we had to complete three and a half academic years then.

Later when I worked in other teaching hospitals and saw some students take their exams repeatedly or leave of their own accord, I would think of Jane. She would have made an excellent physio but on the other hand, I'm sure she eventually made a first rate teacher, it was in her genes.

CHAPTER TWENTY-THREE

Windermere

Sometime early in our final year, we were informed that during the following week we would be going on an educational visit to a long stay hospital for children, in Windermere.

'Sounds like a good day out' I said to Fiona as we read the memo on the notice board. 'It will certainly make a change, I don't think I can stomach much more of the Chest Clinic.'

Poor Fiona, by some quirk of fortune she had done a longer spell than usual at The Chest Unit down the road and as she graphically put it, she was heartedly sick of making people cough and spit. For six weeks she had been treating all manner of chest conditions, asthma, emphysema, chronic bronchitis but mostly cystic fibrosis and bronchiectasis. Bronchiectasis, is usually a congenital condition though it can develop later in life. It is a weakness or under development of the bronchus and the smaller air sacs in the lungs causing secretions to dangerously collect. The patient and their carers, particularly the parents of child patients, have to be taught postural drainage so they can treat the patients every morning and evening, every day, there can be no let up. It is an exhausting procedure both for the patient and the carer. The patient has to be upended, head down feet up, to allow the chest secretions to drain into the main airways. To aid the drainage the therapist has to vigorously shake, clap and vibrate first one lung then the other to allow the patient cough away the secretions. The treatment, as tedious as it is, especially for children, is vital and most patients do feel a whole lot better after their PD, as it is abbreviated to. It is a lifelong commitment and it does impinge on family life, which, as a consequence, does have to be taught well from the beginning.

Getting people to spit seems a bit indelicate and it did take some getting used to. It isn't too bad for the operator if the patient is an accurate spitter, usually a male. Female patients who think it isn't ladylike to spit, which it isn't, do have to be taught that there is no alternative and to just get on with it. Life is just too short for such pretence. Specialist physiotherapists treating chest patients get understandably fed up if not sick, of receiving handfuls of green slime. Of course the most expert are the old male smokers, they spit with accuracy that is a wonder to behold.

So it was no wonder that after nearly two months of all this Fiona was ready for a change.

The day we were to go to the Lake District dawned pleasantly warm and sunny. In fact it was just the right temperature for the hundred mile journey we were to make, crammed as we were, into the hospital mini bus.

There was quite a holiday atmosphere as we drove out of Salford onto the A6, heading for the towns of Chorley, Preston then on to Lancaster. Skirting the Kent estuary, the river emptying into Morcambe Bay, we drove through the glorious countryside of north Lancashire on through the small town of Milnethorpe. In the near distance the lovely foothills of the Lake District were showing as the early morning mist began to lift, giving way to glinting, glorious sunshine. This area of outstanding, natural beauty is where I spent my childhood, so I knew it well.

We continued through Kendal the hills becoming mountains ahead. Through the trees we could see the sun glinting on Lake Windermere on our left. There were boats of various types, people rowing, sailing or taking the ferry. Those of us reared on the author Arthur Ransome, felt like calling, *Swallows And Amazons For Ever.*

We were constantly teased by glimpses of Windermere as we continued north but half way between Bowness and Ambleside we came to a halt. We had stopped at some impressive wrought iron gates at the beginning of a sweeping gravel driveway. The mini bus started up slowly as the gates swung open. We proceeded down the drive, with the gravel spitting up sideways as we scrunched along. There at the bottom of the sweeping approach was a very impressive grand house.

'What a glorious setting for a long stay hospital,' I remarked to Fiona.

'It certainly is different to Salford Royal,' remarked my observant friend.

We swept to a halt outside the huge heavy carved doorway where a woman in a crisply starched uniform stood waiting to greet us.

'Good morning,' the woman said, 'I am Matron. Would you come this way!'

We all trooped in after the Matron into a large common room, which was oak panelled throughout and comfortably furnished. The huge windows went from ceiling almost to the ground but were interrupted lower down by attractive, cosy, cushioned window seats following the curve of the windows. The panoramic views were stunning. The top panes of glass in the splendid windows were of coloured leaded glass but the major part was clear allowing the most breath taking views of the rolling lawns down to the lakeside, across the glinting water of Windermere, to the mountains beyond. To either side of the immaculate lawns were mature trees. There was a majestic cedar of Lebanon, huge arching beech trees and further away, splendid clumps of rhododendrons.

As I gazed at the magnificence of the property, I couldn't help think of the people who had donated this splendid house and land. They must have truly loved children to give all this magnificence for the welfare of children in the North West. 'Just look at the Langdales, I've never seen the Pikes looking so good,' I muttered to my friend.

We toured the wards, which of course had been the reception rooms in the grand house. Today, the rooms seemed a bit sombre for children, the oak panelling had darkened in places and seemed to frown on those not in the sunshine. The children, who were able, were up and about whilst those in bed were busy with activities ranging from schoolwork to painting. It was heartening to see the children who were mobile run and fetch for those confined to bed.

The children for the most part were recovering after orthopaedic surgery and as a consequence were expected to be in hospital for weeks rather than days. There were children in 'frog,' plasters, holding their congenitally unstable hip joints in place until the ball and socket of the hip joint had developed deeper. There were children with scoliosis or crooked backs of various types and degrees, spina bifida, where the vertebral column had not completely fused round the spinal cord. There were some cerebral palsy patients who also had corrective surgery, in fact the whole gambit of congenital conditions was here.

We walked around the beds chatting to the children admiring their paintings and crafts. One little girl, probably about six, who was up and about, slipped her hand in mine and introduced me to the little patients in their beds. There were six or eight beds to a ward, depending on the size of the room and each ward had two assistant nurses and a qualified nurse who was 'Sister.'

We toured the glorious gardens we had seen from the wards. Down at the bottom of the extensive rolling lawn, at the water's edge, was a boathouse, which I couldn't help but peep into. Somehow I was unreasonably disappointed to find it empty, there was no sailing boat tucked away, not even a rowing boat and I turned away to re-join my friends chatting in the sunshine.

Continuing the guided tour, we were shown into the small dining room. There on the refectory table was laid out a delicious spread. There were mounds of dainty sandwiches, small homemade cakes and two enormous fruit cakes of the sort my mother called 'cut and come again cakes.' 'A veritable feast' remarked Fiona and I agreed, I was starving hungry and dying for a cup of tea.

As we were finishing the delicious repast, Miss Bently, our anatomy lecturer who had accompanied us on our trip, rose to thank the matron and her staff for the warm welcome and lovely tea, which we all had so heartily enjoyed. The matron looked suitably gratified as we all joined in with an enthusiastic round of applause.

We trooped out of doorway thanking the matron again as we left and before climbing into the minivan for the journey home, I took a last look, or so I thought, at The Ethel Headley orthopaedic hospital for children at Windermere.

As we drove away, we listened to Paula going all dreamy over treating very small children. It was definitely going to be her speciality she said 'and who knows I might work here as it isn't a million miles from my home in Barrow.'

'Seems reasonable' we all agreed,

'provided she doesn't land herself with a brace of her own first,' whispered my ever cryptic friend.

It was heart breaking for both parents and the children to have to spend so long in hospital away from each other. Visiting was restricted to Wednesday afternoon and the weekends to allow the parents to get to Windermere. It's beautiful location was some compensation for the children perhaps, but it's very location made visiting difficult for the parents living any distance away, as most did.

Two hours later, we were back in sooty, bustling Salford, minus Fiona who had been dropped off in Chorley, as we passed through her hometown. It must have been the first time in nearly three years she had been home before six o'clock.

CHAPTER TWENTY-FOUR

Non Accidental Injury

Nothing quite knocked me back as seeing a child suffering from a non-accidental injury.

Before I had children of my own, I assumed I related with them generally but that in the main I could take them or leave them. For the most part, I left them. At the time, I hadn't any young relatives, none of my friends were married, far less had children and socially I did not come across children generally and certainly not those of tender years.

One morning soon after our trip to Windermere, I was working on the wards and entered 'women's surgical,' and found to my surprise a cot in the centre of the ward. The cot was standing in that unlikely place, complete with its disconsolate looking occupant, because when the child was admitted in the middle of the night there had been absolutely no other place to put this small patient. Susan was her name, a plain ginger haired little girl whose lack of apparent beauty was not enhanced either by her sour expression or her nasty rash around her mouth. At that stage I had not read her case notes but guessed Susan was about three years old but she could have been older. It was difficult to judge, as she was anything but bonny.

'Hello' I said, resting my hands on the side of her cot, looking at this new arrival. The child responded by turning away as far as she could in her confined space, pressing her white face against the bars of the far corner of her cot.

I stood there awkwardly. Not being used to small healthy, friendly children, I was even less used to sick sulky ones. I let the side of the cot down and knelt down to be at her level. That was better. In my pocket I had a small packet of jelly babies, which a patient had slipped into my pocket earlier. Taking the packet out of my pocket I undid one corner and let four of the jewel coloured sweets slowly drop one by one onto her cot cover. Susan stared at them for quite a while, not speaking or moving. I pretended to read her case notes, which I had picked up. Bit by bit a little hand moved out to where the jelly babies lay, then quick as a flash, the sweets were snatched and tucked away in the far corner. 'It's alright Susan they are for you and Sister says you can eat them now if you wish.' For the first time she looked at me, one of the sweets in her fist slowly moving towards her mouth, clearly unsure whether the sweets or herself, were safe.

Susan had been admitted during the night. She had been brought in by a social worker. A neighbour had complained to the police about the 'horrific screaming coming from next door.' When investigations were made, the policewoman had found Susan in agony, along with her distraught mother. Her mother said 'Susan had been playing her up'. Whatever the circumstances, the mother had totally lost control and had sat the child on the hot plate of the cooker. No wonder Susan was half kneeling, half sitting in that peculiar manner, her little bottom was burnt raw.

Although Susan was in the surgical ward *pro tem*, she was in the care of the burns unit and she was soon moved to the specialised ward, where, as it happened, there were two other children. Susan responded well to the treatment, not to mention to rest, regular good food and plenty of cuddles. She soon lost that typical pinched, scared, look such children have. As Susan recovered, she blossomed into an attractive friendly little girl, the rash around her mouth had gone and her red hair had a wonderful shine. Eventually she was discharged into the care of the Local Authority until her mother was able to cope and the child could safely be returned home.

A short time afterwards, I met Paul. He was a skinny, blond lad, thirteen years old. He had been admitted about midnight with extensive cuts and bruising to his legs.

A friend of our family had been returning home after attending a meeting. As she approached her own district, she saw a young boy running wildly down the road. She didn't think much about it at that moment until she had halted at the traffic lights. As she sat there waiting for the lights to change, the boy ran by, he was obviously crying and seemed to be running blindly in any direction without first looking to see if anything was coming. The lights changed and our friend drove on passed the boy then stopped her car. She got out and waited for the youngster to come hurtling by.

Doreen grabbed the boy and tried to steady him before asking him what the matter was. It was some time before the boy could answer, his sobs wracking his whole body as he tried to speak.

'Sit in my car and tell me what is upsetting you so,' said Doreen softly. The boy reluctantly sat in the car and after a while calmed down sufficiently to speak.

'It's my dad, he is mad with me, I don't know why, but he just is and he has started kicking me again.'

'He's kicked you before then?' Asked Doreen.

The boy's eyes welled up again and big tears flowed down his face. He tried to brush them away as he nodded. 'Yes many times, and always when he is wearing his working boots.'

'Let me see your legs, love?' Said Doreen gently.

His bloody legs were swollen to twice the size, full of deep cuts and bright blue new bruises and in between, yellow and brown marks from old fading bruises.

'Where are you running to now?' Doreen quietly continued with her questions. Big tears began to roll again and Doreen put her arms round the lad. 'Just tell me your name?' She asked.

'It's Sam.,' after a while, he added, 'I was going to my granddad's, I usually do, the trouble is my father knows where I'll be.'

'Has this been going on for a long time then?' Asked Doreen gently.

'Yes' was the simple reply.

'Right, I'll drive you to you grandfather's house, you just tell me where he lives OK?' Sam nodded. Without further delay Doreen started the car and guided by her young passenger drove to her new destination. Doreen stopped the car when Sam pointed out the house. 'Don't be afraid, I'll come in with you,' she said. She knocked on the door and a moment later, it was opened by Sam's grandfather. Doreen was about to explain what she was doing there, when the man said 'she had better come in'.

Doreen entered the house and stood close to Sam.

'I don't know why my boy does this to Sam?' the grandfather began sadly. 'He's a good lad and doesn't deserved to be treated this way but I just can't stop my son.'

'Well if you can't stop him I will, I will take Sam to the police station' responded Doreen, causing Sam to weep again.

'You can't do that!' The grandfather said going pale.

'And why not?' Asked our intrepid friend.

'He's a police officer!' Replied the grandfather awkwardly.

'You mean your son is a police officer and is doing this to his own boy?'

The elderly man nodded.

'In that case,' Doreen said, trying to collect her wits 'I'll take Sam with me.'

Doreen drove the boy to the hospital telling the medical staff in A and E what had happened. Once the boy was receiving treatment Doreen rang a friend of hers who was a social worker who arranged an, 'Expedited Place of Safety Order,' with immediate effect. 'Meanwhile Sam's father has been suspended pending an inquiry.'

'And that,' said Doreen when she was relating the horrific story to us all, 'was all I could do.'

We told her in no uncertain terms we thought she was absolutely heroic and was to be congratulated. It was quite coincidental that Sam was allocated to me as my patient for the time he was in hospital and a nicer boy you couldn't hope to meet. Eventually he went to live with his grandfather.

These two children were the first I was to treat for non accidental injuries but by no means the last. Without doubt children are the most vulnerable members of society either being too young to tell others what is happening to them, or often, if the child is older, not knowing to whom to turn and more importantly, who will believe them.

As so often happens I would treat one unusual case only to find another right on its heels.

A week after Sam had been discharged I was given another new patient with a fractured pelvis, with a warning from the Sister to watch out, the rest of the men in the ward are waiting to see your reaction. I looked at her inquiringly but she just shrugged her shoulders and moved off. I pushed open the swing doors of the ward and there in the first bed space in this orthopaedic ward was a cot with a toddler standing up watching for the doors to open. I was the luckless female entering. 'Go away you f****** old witch,' shouted this cherub. All the men patients tried to fix an innocent air as they watched for my reaction. Trying not to break step, I pulled the curtains round the cot to read the child's case notes. Meanwhile the holy terror was repeatedly shouting his request, apparently only applying it to female members of staff. As usual, the child had been admitted in the night, with pain causing his continuous screaming.

The parents were each blaming each other for throwing their child down the stairs. Who ever was to blame, the child had sustained an undisplaced, fracture of his pubic ramus, the bone at the front of his pelvis. Now one can walk with such a fracture and clearly this toddler was doing just that around his cot, so really there was no need for exercises, and considering the high octane expletives that were issuing forth from young Charlie, there was nothing much wrong with his lungs either. The child was too young for school and certainly hadn't been to nursery, so he could only have learnt his choice vocabulary from home. What's more as the blue tirades were always directed at female staff, it certainly made one think about the family relationships the infant was being reared in.

In due course the infant was discharged and the male patients lost a great source of pathetic amusement.

As the evidence was certainly more than sufficient, the child was put on the Child Protection Register when he was discharged.

CHAPTER TWENTY-FIVE

Children's Hospital

As if to remedy my lack of children-related skills, I was sent to do my next stint at the Childrens' Hospital.

The three weeks I was to spend in my first venture into paediatrics, left me with many memories. As I walked into the first ward, there were children, hurrying, scooting, pedalling, laughing, all of whom seemed at first glance, not to be ill at all or incapacitated in any way. These children were aged between three and nine, primary school age I suppose and obviously well on the road to recovery. The children were mostly ready for discharge, and didn't seem to need a physio at that stage anyway.

I entered the next ward, which I found was much quieter with children recovering from having such recent surgery as a tonsillectomy or an appendectomy. There were some children though who had more serious surgery and so at least for the first day post op, peace reigned but wide, watchful eyes followed me around the small wards as I stopped to talk to or treat first one child then another.

The truly remarkable fact about most children, I soon learnt, is their ability to bounce back, one minute they appear desperately ill but the next they are laughing and shouting with the best of them and great to see it is too.

The most harrowing of my small patients were in two categories, the first was those children that had been deliberately hurt. I might not have been the person that Paula was, bibbing and cooing over infants and cots but my job was to reduce pain and to restore a patient, whatever their age, back to full health and pain free. To hurt somebody deliberately, particularly a child, made me feel quite ill and very angry at the same time. I had experienced treating some abused children at the general hospital so I had managed to grow a slight, protective veneer of stoicism, albeit very thin, when I had to treat a child, who had been starved, battered or burnt. Usually all three, but it wasn't easy.

My second harrowing category was, of course, that of the desperately sick child or young person.

When I first met Mike it was obvious he was gravely ill. He had been in hospital many times over the last four years with a variety of leukaemia. At first he responded well to the treatment and after a year or so seemed to have the disease well under control if not beaten.

Mike was eleven years old with bright blue eyes that looked enormous because of his tired face. He had no hair as the result of the chemo that he had to endure, instead he wore a bright woolly hat cheerfully proclaiming his favourite Manchester football team. Round his bed he had numerous photographs of his heroes all of which seemed to carry get well messages along with an autograph and good luck signs.

At first, each morning and afternoon, I would take Mike plus his stand with his drip attached, a short, slow, gentle walk down the corridor and back. It was a much as he could manage and he was always relieved to get back to his bedside chair although he didn't say so. He just pretended the walk was a 'doddle,' and I went along with the pretence but we both knew it was no such thing.

Mike didn't say much a he walked, the effort of it all took all his strength but once back in his chair and rested he told me about his family and school. He was the younger of two sons and he had a black Labrador dog called Pepper he thought the world of and who thought the world of him. Although he had missed a lot of school, over the last couple of years the teachers had been very supportive tailoring his lessons to the time available. His friends at school were equally supportive and regularly sent him get well cards and newsletters full of what was happening in and around school, just letting Mike know he was still part of his class and the world outside.

'But,' said Mike one afternoon with amazing tranquillity, 'I know I won't be able to go back to school, my treatment isn't working anymore.' He paused for a moment. 'I have asked to go home and the doctors have said I can in two days' time.' He looked at me and then continued. 'I am so tired of hospitals and painful treatments, I just want to be with my mum and dad and Harry and especially Pepper my dog, I just miss them all so much.'

It would have been insulting to Mike to try to dismiss what he was telling me in his own matter of fact way, with some flip cheery remark from me. He needed to talk, to be listened to, quietly, with a hand holding his. He needed and received a long hug from me. It was absolutely futile to tell this brave boy he had a future and all was well when it patently wasn't. Mike knew, with absolute certainty, the gravity of his situation and that he was dying. Around his face he had a serenity that seemed to enfold him in the most profound way.

It was an absolute agony for his parents and his older brother, who could only stand by and watch quite helpless in the most heart breaking way. It seemed to me then, that Mike aged eleven, had an inner strength, which, combined with his matter of fact acceptance of his imminent death, was a comfort to his family. In fact it appeared he was supporting them, rather than they supporting him, all of which, as a helpless observer, I found excruciatingly moving.

Mike went home, to the comfort of his home life and his loving family and died tranquilly, four weeks later.

It was difficult not to take tragedy home on some days but I was to learn that children themselves are a lesson in resilience both in life and death and in their very own way, quite inspirational – particularly so with gravely ill children. I found there were many happy and triumphant moments when for example after many weeks a child could stand and walk unaided again, when stitches were removed and smiles broke out, the unmitigated joy of being able to have a good scratch when a plaster cast was removed and the filthy casing complete with many autographs, held up in triumph.

The time I spent at the hospital for children flashed by and yet, in some ways, the three weeks I had spent there seemed like forever. I had seen and learnt a great deal that was new and a great deal that was vaguely familiar but long forgotten. It was a happy and fulfilling, yet sometimes, an exhausting and a sad experience but one not ever to be forgotten.

CHAPTER TWENTY-SIX

More Departures

I was always glad to return to base and the friendly common room. I was looking forward to seeing Fiona again and catching up with all the news. I thought how lucky I was to be meeting up again with good friends, to see the comforting size of Barbara, the white toothy smile of Paula and to join in with the cheery laugh of Sylvia.

So it was with a great deal of pleasure and anticipation I found myself back the following Monday morning. I laughed to myself as I recognised my pleasure, how different had been my journey two and a half years ago when I had so reluctantly dragged myself back to re-join the physiotherapy scene.

More and more, in our final year, we were sent to specialised hospitals and units to gain invaluable experience often for the first time and sometimes for the last. It went without saying that some specialities were more popular than others. The Skin Hospital was never top of the popularity pole at first glance although once there, it was totally different and consequently very interesting. For the most part we all breathed a sigh of relief on our return from the geriatric hospital particularly if we had been confined to the unit for dementia. That work is truly vocational, we all agreed. Where ever we went and however interesting we had found the work, it was always good to return to the fold and compare notes and catch up on the news.

Such a great deal seemed to have happened while I had been away. The strange student who had joined us mid-term from another part of the country had been whisked away with anorexia nervosa.

This student had been at our school for only a few weeks when she decided to have her nose 'corrected.' For weeks afterward she would gaze critically at her profile for what seemed like hours, in front of the one and only mirror in the place, looking for imperfections.

'Quite honestly, I don't see any difference between the before and the afterwards nose, do you?' I asked Fiona one day as we watched the now regular scrutiny of her face.

'Mmm, the difference is certainly minimal considering the probable expense involved,' agreed Fiona.

It seemed whatever inner doubts she might have had about herself, having her nose altered had not helped. She went on a strict diet. We would watch with fascination as she carefully boiled herself a tomato on the one ring cooker, which we had. The ritual continued as she carefully lifted the tomato out of the pan and placed it on a plate. She then took it over to the corner table to eat it like a person in a trance in a slow motion film. Even when she must have weighed not much more than six stone she kept on with her boiled tomato diet.

Some days later, it occurred to me I had not seen this student around in the last couple of days. When I asked if anyone had seen her recently, Barbara announced she had collapsed on one of the wards, she just wasn't strong enough to do anything at all, let alone physio. Bo must have given her a talking-to, because she seems to have moved out lock, stock and barrel. Barbara shrugged her shoulders as she finished telling us the sad saga and for a moment we all sat there inwardly digesting the awful implications of this latest piece of news.

In my brief absence, another daughter of physiotherapy had left these Victorian portals – pregnant. It was a day or two before I realised she was missing from the common room.

'Where's Edna I haven't seen her around for a while?' I asked Paula.

'She has had to leave, of course, as you have been elsewhere you would not have heard.' Paula proceeded to tell me about Edna's fall from grace.

'It seems it was a holiday romance!' Explained Paula. 'what was really grim was the fact that the man was married and Edna didn't know.' She continued. 'When Edna told him about the baby he just pushed off, he didn't want anything to do with her.'

'Oh Lord,' I muttered.

'There was talk about someone who could supply the right sort of pills,' said Paula, as she lowered her voice to barely a whisper.

'My goodness she will kill herself if she tries anything like that!' I whispered back, horrified. Abortion was illegal then and all of us students had seen the results of septic abortions by that stage in our careers.

'Nobody in their right mind would contemplate a seedy room in a back street and all the terrible risk that went with such a grim venture,' I said as Sylvia who had came over and stood listening to the conversation about

Edna's predicament.

'The thing is she probably is out of her mind with worry and trying to think of all the possible options,' I added, and both Paula and Sylvia nodded.

'I don't know what Bo said to her when she went to see her but I found Edna here after she had been to the office, packing up her things,' said Sylvia

It was the first any of us had heard about it. I think she has resigned herself to having the baby, but I couldn't help but feel sorry for Edna, she never had been one of us, always seemingly to choose to be by herself in so many ways. I knew she was an only child and her parents were quite elderly.

'I wonder how her parents are taking the news?' I asked. Nobody knew for certain but the feeling was that she was at home and her parents were standing by their daughter.

It was a measure of the tragedy, as it was seen in those days, that even Paula, the one who went into a happy delirium at the thought of babies, was visibly shaken.

CHAPTER TWENTY-SEVEN

Mary

On a more cheerful note Fiona's sister had become engaged. Mary was also a physiotherapist who had qualified a year previously and was now working at the general hospital in her hometown.

Mary's fiancé sounded quite amazing and we listened with growing envy as she described this veritable answer to a maiden's prayer. He was, it seemed, a tall, handsome solicitor by profession with a promising future in local government. To crown all the obvious attributes, Robert had the wonderful bonus of being able to both design a dress and then make it. Totally untaught, he would buy Mary some exquisite material, sit down at his mother's sewing machine and run up a fabulous gown. Nor did his talent end there, anything that Mary required, be it a suit or a day dress, all she need do it seemed, was to express her requirements and lo and behold there it was. Fiona sat there and continued to extol her future brother-in-law's many talents whilst we hung on every word.

'Some girls have all the luck, man, money and what a talent,' said Barbara echoing all our sentiments.

Mary was attractive and strong willed, given to expletives if she thought the situation of the moment warranted it. One memorable evening, prior to the appearance of Robert her intended, she had been out with some pukka chap when a particular incident had occurred which she felt, merited, 'oh the bugger.' 'The pukka gentleman did not appreciate this from his lady friend apparently,' related Fiona as she sipped her coffee.

'What happened then?' I said, riveted by the turn of the conversation. Actually I was about to return to the wards leaving half my drink unfinished but picking up my cup I quickly sat down again.

'Well this fellow took her aside and informed her if they were to continue going out together she had better modify her vocabulary'. Mary was suitably admonished, no small feat considering her temperament 'but,' continued Fiona, 'Mary was pretty keen on this chap, at the time, or she would have told him where to go so she looked for and found another expletive which she felt would give vent to her feelings but not embarrassment to the sensitive gentleman.'

'The next time this chap came calling,' continued Fiona, 'was to take Mary to a very smart party. During the course of the evening, some clown spilt his drink all down the front of Mary's dress. This was all Mary needed to trigger her new found expression, 'oh balls,' she said, her clear voice hanging about the room like early morning mist. Most of the guests present pretended not to hear, the rest looked amused to varying degrees.'

'Then what happened?' I asked Fiona.

'Well Mary's chap seemed most embarrassed and was seething mad but there was nothing he could do except try to mop up the spilt wine. Anyway, how was she to know that balls were testicles,' concluded Fiona, in her sister's defence.

How indeed, educated as they were at their convent, when even taking their night time bath they were advised to wear an all covering shift so the sight of their own body did not cause offence.

Fiona was still seeing her lanky, big footed, large Adam's apple, of good family type fellow. She wasn't actually admitting to boredom because as she put it, 'he did hunt and so she couldn't complain.'

'How's your social life?' she asked.

'About the same,' I answered. 'I seem to have got myself into a pleasant and comfortable rut. I don't go out during the week because Roland works out of town but life seems to consist of going to the university hop on Saturday night and going out for the day on Sunday, walking in the countryside.'

'Sounds alright,' said Fiona.

'Well I can't deny it isn't pleasant, it is. It is lovely being taken out and being looked after. I suppose if I'm honest, I feel I'm being settled down and I am not ready for that yet. I am not ready for marriage and although he has not mentioned it, I know that is what he wants. What is complicating the scene,' I continued, 'is that now we always end up at his parents' house for an evening meal on Sunday nights. They are lovely people but I do feel the matrimonial noose tightening.' I had been subconsciously counterbalancing the undeniable pleasure and reassurance of Roland's company, with the vague, uneasy thought that one day, I might end up on the shelf.

Fiona listened sympathetically, in some measure I was only reflecting her own thoughts in relation to her 'of good family' chap.

'I feel a bit guilty by still going out with him when I know he wants to marry me.' I went on, sitting there unburdening myself to my friend. 'He hasn't actually asked me yet but when the conversation veers that way, I have tried to explain to him how I feel. I have told him I don't want to take advantage of him but he just laughs it off, he seems to think time will change my mind. I just feel as if I'm in some pleasant emotional quick sand,' I finished lamely.

'Don't worry, it will probably fizzle itself out,' said Fiona.

I nodded, grateful for the sympathy, but still full of doubt.

I certainly wanted to get married some time but not then. Indeed, I was looking forward immensely to the day when I was qualified and could support myself. It seemed somehow or other I was subconsciously absorbing pressures in society in general and in the students common room in particular. Some of the girls were now engaged and busy planning for their big day. Then of course there was Roland.

The pressure was definitely not coming from my parents. My father was slightly old fashioned as far as daughters and matrimony were concerned He certainly thought his daughter should marry but didn't actually say as much. However, he did emphatically believe in equal rights for women. My mother though, was all for independence and higher education. 'Only being an independent person in your own right will you find true happiness,' my mother was to tell me from time to time. She was right.

CHAPTER TWENTY-EIGHT

Tennis, Tans and Holidays

With summer fast approaching, the tennis fanatics began to show themselves. Each lunch time, four or possibly six, of our number grabbed their tennis racquets and headed for Peel Park. At least two of the girls had reached county championship level in their final year at school and they led the lunchtime charge. Out they ran, not a moment to spare, as indeed there wasn't, as they had to dash round the Crescent, the big arc of the River Irwell, to get to the public tennis courts in the Salford park. Mercifully our immediate group were not smitten by the craze. Sylvia said 'she didn't know where they got the energy from, it was not as if we were typists and desk bound'.

Instead of this hectic tennis campaign, we decided that as the holidays were approaching we would steal a march on our friends and treat ourselves to a course of ultra-violet light to get ourselves a tan. Although it was a treatment we often administered to patients, we were forbidden to treat ourselves without going through the formalities of getting permission from a qualified staff member.

Actually, we rarely treated anybody with a general dose of UVL. Long gone were the days of treating rickets both in children and adults or giving miners 'sunlight' to counter their work underground. We treated cases such as leg ulcers, bedsores, arthritis and severe acne. Doses were always carefully recorded and monitored so the next physio to treat the patient would know exactly what dose had been given and how much the dosage was to be progressed next time. In some treatments specialised filters were required to cut out unwanted rays for a particular condition but for both the patient and the member of staff, we always protected the eyes, without this, you were liable to get severe conjunctivitis or worse.

Regardless of the threatened penalties for treating ourselves, the five of us would slip away and give ourselves a course of 'sunlight.' We took great care not to cook each other but I don't expect we fooled the staff. Anyone, who has any experience of UVL, could spot an artificial erythema or pinking of the skin a mile off.

If it was obvious to the staff we were treating ourselves, and it must have been, then it was equally obvious to us we were being ignored. We were only months off qualification and were deliberately keeping our treatments low key. We certainly did not want the pain and discomfort of sunburn, nor did we want to look grey and wrinkled days later not to mention peeling in strips before the week was out.

Merrill, a strong, olive skinned, athletic girl in our year had been treating herself to some UVL, for some time, to try to counter the tendency to spots, caused she thought, by her slightly oily skin.

Returning from holiday, the march that she had stolen on her non-physio friends in getting a head start in the sun tan department, somewhat backfired as she came back through passport control, causing them huge amusement and her great indignation. The group had been to the Italian Riviera and on her return to this green and pleasant land she was stopped by a chap in uniform, an immigration official. He wanted to know where she was going in England and what her business was once she had arrived at her destination. She replied indignantly 'that she was born in England and she was bred in Eccles, of cake fame.' Further 'she was returning home to finish her studies and she would be obliged if he would let her pass without any more delay or she would be late for work at Salford Royal Hospital.'

The Official rechecked her passport then handing her documents back, apologised as he did so, explaining his behaviour by adding English girls didn't usually turn that colour in two weeks even in Italy. I don't recollect Merrill giving herself any more courses of 'sunlight' prior to future holidays.

We had four weeks holiday in the summer not a long time compared with other unpaid students and far too short a time for any potential employer to be interested in us. Most of us were broke of course and some holiday job would have been welcome to help the coffers but it wasn't to be. In a way it was a good thing, we worked physically hard as well as studying hard so just to have a change away was what we needed.

I had to decide how best to spend these precious four weeks. I was broke so there was no thought of holidays abroad. Last year a friend and I had a walking holiday exploring the Yorkshire coast. We had started at Bridlington and walked north for the next ten days, through Filey, round Flamborough Head to Scarborough. We continued on to Whitby, via the stunning Robin Hood's bay ending up at the gentle town of Saltburn. It had been hard going at first until we literally got into our stride but all along the coast was beautiful and new to us and we were lucky with the weather. Trying to get into our stride with aching feet and sore shoulders from our rucksacks reminded me of the words of one of my patients. As it happened he had once been in the French Foreign Legion and during one of our interesting conversations about the rigours of that life he had said probably anyone could walk forty miles in a day but not too many could walk forty miles day after day especially over difficult terrain, it definitely sorted the men from the boys. As I was aching everywhere and not walking anything like forty miles a day, I was feeling very much a 'boy' at that moment. But that was last year.

Suddenly the coming four weeks became action packed. Another walking friend asked me if I would join her exploring the Quantocks. To be honest I wasn't quite sure where the Quantock hills were but then that sounded as good a reason as any, to go and find out. So off we went, starting at Bristol. We hugged the coast almost as far as Watchet then turned southeast, walking in beautiful gentle countryside. We stayed in lovely villages before going north through Glastonbury back to catch the train at Bristol. Here again we were lucky with the weather, which was just as well, getting into one's stride takes a day or two and being repeatedly wet through would have definitely taken the edge off our regional safari.

Then it was back home for a night before going north to a small village west of Carlisle where I was to be an unpaid helper at a Summer School. I knew the place well, for years ever since I was old enough, I had spent a week there and had enjoyed the greatest fun. When I was asked if I might help out on the staff I was only too pleased to do so hoping I could help to give back some of the fun I had shared and received over the years. The weather was mixed but it didn't matter it was the greatest fun and the week flew by.

I returned to Manchester with only a couple of days to get my things washed and packed before I joined my parents and younger brother on a family holiday in the Lake District. We were staying at a place, which was well known to us, and it was very comforting to know we would have a great time there. The views and walks were fantastic and the homemade food quite delicious and plentiful. We had a wonderful time and promised as usual to return whenever we could.

The four precious weeks were up and time to return to the grindstone. I felt as if I had been away much longer than I actually had, probably due to the fact I'd had such a delightfully busy time. I felt refreshed both mentally and physically and ready for the remaining few weeks that were left before my final examinations. I could not believe the past three years had flown by so quickly and that already the end was in sight.

CHAPTER TWENTY-NINE

Vote of Confidence

Suddenly the summer was over and I found myself back in the familiar routine of being up early and out of the door running to the bus stop, heading for the centre of Manchester and on to Salford, in one frantic dash.

As I arrived at the hospital, the common room was buzzing with greetings and laughter as tales of holidays were exchanged. Everyone seemed glad to be back in the comforting atmosphere of our friends warm companionship This was our last term and, amongst us, there were mixed of feelings of uncertainty and anxiety as to what the future would hold and we were conscious of the fact this would be the last time we would meet up together after our holidays, like this.

We were busy getting into our uniforms when someone called to me and said Bo wanted to see me at once. I hadn't been back at the hospital for an hour when the summons came and as I hurried to Bo's office, I wondered what was afoot. All sorts of thoughts went through my mind as I approached her door, I couldn't think there was a problem, any way I certainly hoped that was the case. I knocked on the office door and listened for the call.

'Enter,' was the imperious summons, and I opened the door.

'Ah Miss Arden come in and sit down,' Bo said. I drew up a chair and sat down looking at my boss across her desk. 'Do you remember the Children's' Orthopaedic Hospital which a group of you visited in June?' She said, wasting no time.

I nodded.

'Well,' continued Bo 'the physiotherapist in charge there would like to go to The International Congress which starts next week and she is having difficulty in finding a suitable locum to cover her absence. Would you consider taking on the post?' She looked searchingly at me.

I was quite stunned. In the immediate silence that followed her startling request I tried to gather my wits. Bo has asked me out of all the students both male and female available, to do this. It was without doubt an honour to be asked after all I was still a student albeit a final year one. What is more I would be working on my own with no other physiotherapist to call on.

'The locum post will be for a period of two weeks,' Bo continued, while all the implications were flashing through my mind. 'And to enable you to get there in plenty of time you should arrive the day before. You will live at the hospital and naturally you will be paid.'

The word rang through my mind loud and clear, 'paid,' yet it seemed of secondary importance. I had been without money for the last three years, I could certainly manage a bit longer. No! what was important to me was the fact I knew Bo would not have asked me to go if she thought I could not do the job. I was grateful for her undoubted confidence in me and although I did not say as much, I felt it a point of honour to take the locum post. I would do it, not for the salary nor for the unknown Miss Hepplethwaite, the resident physiotherapist, but for Bo. I had to go and I had to do my best, for her. Bo was that sort of person.

'Most certainly I will go and thank you very much for asking me Miss Bodoano.'

'Good,' Bo smiled briefly before continuing. 'Of course your final examinations are only two months away. If you would prefer to stay here, I do understand but quite honestly, I think you will gain a great deal of useful experience in those two weeks which can only be of the greatest value in the exams and in your future work.'

'I should like to go' I nodded my agreement, 'I should like to go very much' I reassured her.

'Good,' she beamed, 'I am sure you will have no problems.'

As Bo stood up, I pushed my chair out of the way and stood up too, fervently hoping she was correct in her 'no problems,' optimism.

Over coffee I told Fiona why Bo had sent for me. 'I hope I'm doing the right thing.'

'Of course you are, Bo would not have asked you to go if she were in any doubt, I would take the whole trip as one great vote of confidence in you' my friend retorted. Soon the news was round the common room. There seemed to be a mixture of responses from, 'why her?' To 'hearty congratulations, and on being paid too!'

My parents were pleased for me. They too saw it as a vote of confidence in me, and my abilities but they did express some reservation when they realised how near it was to my finals; over all though they thought it 'a very good thing.'

That Saturday night, at the university dance, I told Roland I was to go to the hospital in Windermere for two weeks beginning next Sunday. I knew Roland was definitely the sort of person who would question the advisability of his girlfriend going anywhere for two weeks without him although I could see that he too thought my being asked, was indeed a bit special.

The following Sunday evening I caught the train to Windermere. Roland had driven me to the station carrying my case along the platform. As I approached the train he said he would be drive up to Windermere first thing next Saturday morning and would book himself into a hotel. With that the train pulled out of the station and swept round the big curving bend leaving both of us waving until Roland was out of sight.

I closed the window and sat down in the corner seat of an empty compartment. Clearly not many people were travelling to Windermere at five o'clock on a Sunday evening.

As I made myself comfortable, a great feeling of independence swept over me. The totally new sensation of freedom and liberty filled me with light-hearted joy. As the train picked up speed, I sat there watching the scenery zapping by. I thought of Roland and his plans to visit me next weekend and a slight feeling of suffocation marred my sense of freedom. Suddenly my unlimited, glorious horizon was curbed, defined like a black edged Victorian funeral card. I sat there glumly for a moment or two, trying not to think of The Ethel Headly Children's Orthopaedic Hospital at all.

Suddenly, I came to, cheer up I told myself briskly who knows you might be jolly glad to see him by next weekend. I thought of the serious sum of seven pounds for each of the two weeks, equal to the basic pay a newly qualified physio would receive and additionally of course, I was getting my keep. It was not a great deal of money even then but to someone totally without financial means, it was a princely sum.

Considerably cheered by now, I thought of the delightful house and how glorious the countryside would be in the middle of September. The weather was set fair promising to be an Indian summer. Everything it seemed would be at its very best and with the promise of delicious food too. With that comforting thought, I snuggled back into my corner seat.

As the train moved steadily north, I could see the mountains of the Lake District faintly in the distance. Beyond the town of Carnforth, where they had filmed the great movie *Brief Encounter*, on through Warton and Silverdale, the train sped

Over the nearby hill and out of sight now that the old wooden clock tower had been removed, was the village of Yealand where I had lived and played as a child. As I saw the familiar countryside, my gratitude to Bo swept over me in overwhelming bouts. Her confidence in me had in turn given me confidence in myself.

I smiled as I remembered the reaction of all my friends when I had told them the news. They had been as incredulous as me when I told them word for word what Bo had said. Barbara, ever mindful of the inner man, had reminded everyone of the sumptuous tea that had been plentifully laid out before us on our visit. 'Do you remember those mountains of cakes and other goodies, you are a lucky thing,' then looking at her watch groaned, 'oh God, there's another hour to lunch'. Good old Barbara I thought as I relaxed back into the train seat and put my feet up.

CHAPTER THIRTY

A Different Windermere

The train drew into the station with the porter calling out, 'Windermere, Windermere.' I gathered up my things, there was no desperate hurry, the train went no further, this was the end of the line. Clutching my bag and case I struggled to pull down the leather strap to open the door window. It was impossible to move. I put down my bags and now with two hands free I gave the leather strap a mighty wrench and this time it worked and the window in the door opened. Just as I was putting my hand through the open window to open the carriage door the porter beat me to it. I stepped down from the train and joined the one or two people heading for the ticket barrier. Bo had told me arrangements had been made for me to be met at the station and as the station looked pretty deserted I was very relieved to know this.

Yes, 'that must be Doctor Oxford standing there looking purposefully at me, it couldn't be anybody else,' I told myself. Although I had never met the doctor before it was obvious that she was waiting for someone and as I was the only person about by now, it had to be me.

'Miss Arden?' She said unhesitatingly, extending her hand as I stepped through the barrier. We shook hands.

'Yes, I'm Betsy Arden, how do you do?'

'I don't think we've met,' Dr Oxford continued, 'I'm Dr Oxford and my car is over there.'

'Thank you,' I nodded as she pointed towards her car, 'and thank you for meeting me.'

'The buses are so infrequent, it really is the only way and anyway I wasn't doing anything in particular.' She explained without any accent with a quiet voice that was in keeping with her modest appearance.

What a very pleasant person, I thought warming to her at once. She was tall, thin and angular, about five eight, with greying hair. I guessed her to be nearly sixty but she could have been less after all I was looking at her from a twenty-one-year-old's perspective. The doctor was definitely a country sort of person everything she wore reflected that. She was wearing a brownish Harris Tweed suit, sturdy brown brogues and a brown pull on cloche hat that was straight out of the nineteen twenties.

'Here we are,' she said as we turned the corner. Standing there was the most substantial, elegant, black sedan car parked by the roadside. We put my things into the boot then I joined her in the front. We glided from the kerb in the most luxurious silence. I wondered how long ago it had been since I had seen a privately owned black car. There were city taxis in Manchester, funeral directors and of course the Lord Mayor had a large black car but I couldn't think of any ordinary motorist with such an imposing vehicle.

'This is my parents' car,' she said having read my thoughts. 'They have a chauffeur and my mother thinks it only appropriate that he drives a black car.' She continued with a smile as we sped along the deserted road; it lit up her face, shattering her sombre image. 'My parents are elderly,' she continued as we bowled along, 'and they don't hold with the new garish colours as they put it.' I was laughing as she told me about her people, what a super person I thought and how very pleasant it was travelling in this stately manner.

Half way between Windermere and Ambleside, we slowed down and turned into the driveway. In the twilight, I hadn't recognised it until we had actually made the turn, the entrance coming so immediately after a sharp bend. Yes there we were, the limestone chippings spitting up against the wheels of the car just as I remembered them. The drive looked dark and sombre now, the rhododendrons seemingly closing in as they cut out the last of the day's light. As we swept up to the front door I could glimpse the gunmetal sheen on the lake through the trees.

'Here we are,' she said, bringing the car to a halt 'I'll just ring the bell for Sister in charge then leave you to it.' The doctor stepped up to the heavy wooden door and rang the bell while I collected my bags from the car boot. The door opened after a few seconds and there stood a small woman in a navy dress and starched white apron,

'Good evening doctor,' she said.

'This is Miss Arden,' the doctor said, introducing me, 'the locum physiotherapist. Will you look after her please?'

'I must be getting back now,' Doctor Oxford said turning to me. 'I look forward to seeing you tomorrow, soon after nine.'

I thanked her again and she just smiled and brushed my thanks aside with a little gesture of her hand.

Sister Bedford did not make a habit of smiling. 'If you will follow me I will show you to your room,' she said in a somewhat detached way. Picking up my case, I followed her thinking that this native was not of the particularly friendly type. Small, thin, middle aged, Sister Bedford wasted no time in wondering whether or not I could manage my cases as she set off at a brisk pace. Down a short corridor we went, up a narrow stone staircase, which I registered, was of the servants' type, onto a landing before turning down a further short corridor.

'Bathroom, lavatory, storeroom,' Sister Bedford tapped on the various doors as we hurried past. She did not bother to open any of the doors far less check I was at her heels. She finally halted at a door at the end of the corridor and flinging it open marched in. 'I think you will find this adequate,' Sister Bedford said, looking at me for the first time, with her hands clasped primly in front of her apron.

The room was not overly furnished. It contained a hospital-type bed, typically black in colour, a battered chest of drawers and a small wooden chair. Looking at the Sister, I said

'Yes it is adequate.' I said, looking at the Sister. I deliberately repeated her word but gave it a small degree of enthusiasm that I certainly wasn't feeling. I went to the window, well not so much as went, I was already there, in this small room. In the gathering dusk I could see there was a very limited view of the garden and none whatsoever of the lake.

Sister Bedford switched on the light at the doorway, which only gave me a better view of the limited accommodation. The floor was covered in old-fashioned linoleum, of an indeterminate colour and next to my bed a narrow rug that had certainly seen better days.

With the lights switched on, it seemed pitch black outside and Sister Bedford drew the sad looking curtains together. As she closed the skimpy material, the folds straightened out showing wide, dense, black seams of hibernating bluebottles. As she disturbed the curtains so she disturbed the flies. Suddenly the air was black with sleepy buzzing bluebottles so dizzy that they were flying into everything including themselves and worse, us. I felt quite sick as I tried to avoid being dive bombed. In seconds the flies came to, the whole room was now alive with a furious buzzing and disgusting thuds as the flies hit the windows and us, at speed.

'I'd better go and get a fly spray,' announced my guide and spinning on her heel, the chilling woman disappeared.

I turned to the sash window and tried to lift the bottom section, it just would not budge. I heaved on the top part that was equally stuck. It must have been many years since the window was opened and judging from the hundreds of flies buzzing around in their indignant manner, the sun-bleached curtains had lain undisturbed for the same amount of time.

I walked to the door peering down the corridor, refusing to stay in that disgusting room. 'Where is that wretched female,' I asked myself out loud. I moved the chair into the corridor and sat down waiting for her return. As I sat there I was reminded of my childhood and the corny joke my Manchester born, father once told me.

'Where do all the flies go in winter?' he had asked me, and in true pantomime manner I had asked,

'Where do all the flies go in winter?' and he replied gleefully

'Through Denton to Hyde.' Wrong, they go to Windermere, I thought ruefully.

Sister Bedford eventually arrived back on the scene with the only thing she could find, a small spray no bigger than a man's thumb, of local anaesthetic. She aimed the small container in the general direction of the curtains and gave a few short bursts. That only disturbed the bluebottles again as they had taken the opportunity to settle themselves once more in the Sister's long absence. The angry flies zoomed and buzzed apparently immune to the spray, which is more than I could say for myself. Then gradually the crazed flies began dropping out of the sky as it were. They were falling everywhere. The nightmare took a new turn, not only were the flies falling fast and furiously onto the bed where I was supposed to sleep but they were dropping on to our heads and into our hair.

Feeling decidedly ill by now I was not in the least comforted when Sister Bedford said, 'well there we are, you will be alright now, see you at supper, its seven o'clock sharp in the dining room.' She closed the door after her, glad no doubt, to be beating a hasty retreat.

I couldn't believe she could just go, leaving me with the resulting nightmare. I surveyed the room. The flies were dying noisily. Bluebottles totally covered the counterpane. There were bluebottles buzzing and noisily spinning on their backs on the windowsill and on the linoleum. Only one or two remained airborne, flying in circles around the dingy light bulb. I carefully picked up the four corners of the bed cover and shook the contents carefully into a pile in the corner of the room. I then rolled up the little bedside rug and using it as a brush swept all the rest of the disgusting flies away to join their dead brethren. When all the surfaces were cleared, I grabbed my sponge bag and towel and headed for the bathroom. I felt decidedly unclean and I thought I only hope I can sleep tonight.

I felt better after a good wash and brush up and cheered myself up with the thought that at least the food was good at this place. 'Right here goes, now for the dining room,' I told myself. It was not difficult to find. I entered the small oak panelled room, containing a refectory table and eight matching oak chairs. There were four places set and as I entered, I saw I was the last to arrive, not a good start. Two of the Sisters were in uniform, the third was in 'mufti.' She was resident at the hospital but obviously was not on duty.

As it was such a small hospital, everyone who was actually qualified as a state registered nurse, was automatically elevated to the rank of Sister. The rest of the nursing staff, were in fact, nursing assistants who lived in the surrounding districts.

I smiled as I entered and said, 'good evening.' The response was not exactly ebullient, just a nod and a polite,

'good evening.' As I drew my chair up I looked at the three women, all of whom must have been in their late fifties. Nobody bothered to introduce themselves, so I just smiled and returned their nod.

There seemed nothing to say, no conversation. We all sat with our eyes glued to a plate on the centre of the table. On this lone plate, one thin, slice of shop bought, white bread rested. It was evenly cut into four neat pieces. My drooping spirits dropped completely. There is nothing more telling about what to expect when the meal does eventually arrive than a meagre, miserly breadbasket. Such stinginess always foretells a mean meal. Although still a student, I had worked in seven or eight hospitals on secondment and almost without exception, I had learnt that the better the food the better the hospital was.

The gloomy, silence was broken by the maid pushing open the door and bringing in the pre-poured soup. She carried two bowls, which she placed in front of the two Sisters nearest the door. All eyes turned to examine the contents. The soup rejoiced in the name of, 'brown Windsor.' Whatever its name and there was precious little of it in any case, it reappeared later as gravy.

The meal continued, with a-hard-to-identify slice of meat, boiled potatoes, soggy cabbage and the reinvented gravy. The conversation remained non existent, except for the rare, occasional monosyllabic utterance. As soon as they had finished their Spartan repast, the two Sisters on duty, pushed back their chairs and stood up. They nodded to me and without waiting for the third Sister, hurried off. The third Sister carefully scraped the last vestige of her rice pudding from her dish and deliberately putting her spoon to one side, she too rose to leave.

'Will you be eating your piece of bread?' She suddenly asked as I caught her eye.

'No,' I replied, a bit surprised.

'Then I will take it for later' she said quickly picking up the quarter slice and disappeared from the room.

By this time I was beginning to realise I had volunteered for a stint at a latter day *Do-the-Boys' Hall* to quote Mr Dickens. What was worse, I was beginning to wish that Roland was nearby to bail me out of this miserable situation and it wasn't even my first day technically.

I gloomily pushed my chair back and rose from the table. I was trying to tell myself I was a weak-kneed fool thinking of running into the arms of a man, at the first signs of trouble. It wouldn't have been too bad if I'd had a car supposing I could drive, or even if there had been a bus service that ran more frequently than every other day. There just was no escape. No wonder those physiotherapists wiser than I had not volunteered to take the locum post here. And what a sham that marvellous tea had been on our visit, talk about never judging a book by its cover. With that indignant thought, I returned to my tiny room.

The door was still open, as I had purposely left it. Without actually going into the room, I switched on the light and listened. All seemed to be quiet. Here and there, one or two flies lay on the windowsill and on the counterpane, not as bad as it was but bad enough. I swished them all into the 'dead-fly corner.' Suddenly there was a loud, furious buzzing. I spun round to see a large dying bluebottle, on the floor, whirling about on its back in its frantic death throws. I watched it hypnotised, then, grabbing one of my shoes, killed it and flicked it off to join its dead companions. Ugh, I shuddered.

Never mind things will look a lot better after a good night's sleep I told myself. I opened my suitcase and unpacked my things. At the bottom of my case was my faithful hot water bottle, I never went anywhere without it. I looked at my watch, it was only nine o'clock, even for me, it was a bit early to go to bed. I was definitely a lark. I preferred to go to bed early and be up early rather than the other way round. I had brought a couple of books to read but the light was dim, too poor to read anyway. I made a mental note that come the weekend, when Roland came, I would do a bit of shopping and a light bulb of sufficient strength was on the list along with plenty of edibles.

I went to the bathroom, cleaned my teeth and filled my hot water bottle. Mercifully there was a good supply of hot water so I decided I would soak in the bath before retiring. Having killed another half an hour, I climbed into bed and wrapped myself around my hottie. This might not be a merry haven of lightness and gaiety but tomorrow I will meet the children, perhaps they will be pleased to see me. I pulled the string of the 'lazy Mary,' light switch above my head and snuggled down. Thinking of the children had cheered me up. Thank goodness it was not a unit for dementia I thought. I was quite determined that during the next two weeks, the children and I, were going to not only work hard but enjoy ourselves too.

Much to my surprise, I slept very well but then I always do on very hard beds. I reached for my watch, 'um five past seven just nice time to rise in a leisurely way and not be first in the dining room for breakfast,' I told myself. I climbed out of bed and pattered to the window, the floor was cold under my feet.

The lawn was heavily dewed and there was a hanging mist everywhere. It promised to be another glorious September day. I turned to the chest of drawers and took out one of my folded and well starched, white coats. I shook it open and collected a handful of white buttons and their metal shanks. Sitting on the side of the bed, feet well off the chilly floor, I began to button through my coat.

Popping through to the bathroom, which I gratefully noted nobody else seemed to use, I had a wash and brush up. Five minutes later, I was ready. Clad in my crisp white coat, starched belt wrapped round my twenty one inch waist, I was ready for whatever the day was to bring. Just being in my uniform was reassuring; one became a person in one's own right, with a job to do. In 'mufti,' one was a nonentity, without authority.

Breakfast was no surprise after last night's dinner. 'Good morning,' I said brightly forcing some response. I thought of my mother who could always elicit a 'good morning,' out of the most aloof people if she was so determined. I went to my place and sat down; the pattern was much the same as before. Those on duty gulping down their meal leaving those of us who were left, making sure anything that was edible was either eaten there or 'taken for later.' I wondered if I would be equally, desperately hungry by the end of the week. I hoped not, as come to think of it, I don't remember seeing a shop anywhere near here. I looked at my watch, it was twenty past eight, I was due to meet Doctor Oxford in half an hour. Well there is nothing to keep me here, I told myself and pushing back my chair, stood up and left to clean my teeth.

CHAPTER THIRTY-ONE

My Friends The Children

Soon after breakfast Dr Oxford arrived. She greeted me cordially and asked if I had slept well. I replied in the affirmative, not bothering to tell her about the plague of bluebottles. Together we visited every little ward and I was formally introduced to the Sisters I'd had my meals with previously with the exception of one who had been away for the weekend. This last Sister, a little, plump, grey haired woman, distinguished herself with her cheery friendly smile as we shook hands. I made a note of Sister Jones, up until now there had been a definite dearth of anything approaching a warm welcome other than from Doctor Oxford.

We stopped briefly at each child's bed and had a word with every small patient. The doctor outlined, their condition, the treatment including any surgery the child might have had, how long they had been at this hospital and their prognosis for the future. I made notes as we did the rounds.

'Well now you have met everyone,' said Dr Oxford when we had completed our tour. 'I'll leave you to it, if you have any problems don't hesitate to come to me.' I thanked her and said I certainly would if I needed to. 'Right-ho' She said briskly and we went our different ways.

It was becoming increasingly obvious that it would be impossible to treat all the children individually the first day. I split the children into groups those that needed individual treatment daily, mostly those relatively new to the hospital and probably still confined to bed. Those that were up, I decided, could join me in the tiny physio department or in one of the bigger spaces I had located. I could treat the mobile children in the afternoon by way of exercises disguised as games, always popular. I loved 'remedial class taking,' not all my colleagues thought the same way understandably, but I always had great fun and as far as I was concerned the more the merrier, within reason. With any luck, my patients and I could spend some treatment time with therapy sessions on the lawn, if the weather stayed as it was. It was a shame to waste this late warm sunshine, and I was certain the children would love it.

The first day was hectic. Getting to know my patients, who mostly had congenital conditions like scoliosis or curvature of their back, dislocated hips, which were in frog plasters to hold the hip joints in place until they had corrected themselves, or perhaps severe asthmatics. It was good that the conditions varied it made my work all the more interesting.

At the end of the day I went to my room to lay on my bed until it was time to go down to dinner. I just hadn't realised just how exhausted I was. Effective treatment mostly takes half an hour per patient and often longer. During that time, you had to constantly coax, encourage and sometimes, scold, to get the patients to give of their utmost. Only if they try their best each time can progress be made. Often the progress is infinitesimally slow or slight even after a hard slog. Then, some slight improvement is obtained and like so many other things once started, recovery has a way of escalating.

In addition to my inpatients, I had one out patient who was brought by her mother on a Wednesday afternoon all the way from Grange over Sands, on the northern part of Morecambe Bay. It was a long and difficult journey especially by public transport.

Joya was a pleasant girl, nine-years old who came with her mother, a dark Italian woman. The little girl was born with both hips dislocated. They were dislocated, not by rough treatment, but by both the balls of the hip bones being flattish in shape and because the cups into which the head of femur should have been snugly held, were very shallow. The result was very unstable hips, which would have prevented Joya from learning to walk as an infant.

Conservative treatment had been tried at first when she was a baby, by way of a frog plaster to hold the babies hips in the optimum position but after a year no real improvement was obtained, both hips were still badly unstable. In the end Joya had to have bilateral corrective surgery. The surgery was a great success and originally she had spent some time post operatively as an inpatient here at Windermere. The surgery was a success but the child had suffered muscular weakness after so long in a plaster and she needed regular physiotherapy to try to make up for those vital initial few months in her life.

On leaving the hospital here, Joya and her mother had been shown and given a list of essential exercises the child had to do to improve her mobility, strength and stamina, of her hip and leg muscles. The purpose of this weekly visit was to ensure Joya was doing her exercises and that all was well.

On the second week that Joya attended, she shyly offered me a little gift. Delighted by the kindly thought, I opened the small parcel and found it contained a carton of Morecambe Bay, buttered potted shrimps, delicious.

Joya's mother was Italian, hence the unusual name of her child. The mother had married a local man who had always lived in the Morecambe Bay area. He was a by trade a 'shrimper.' She helped her husband in the business by cooking the shrimps, peeling them and finally packing them into cartons, sealing the delectable contents with melted butter. From their Grange over Sands home they were sent to delicatessens nationwide. The work involved was not only dangerous in the hazardous waters of the Bay but extremely labour intensive. Joya's father worked all hours and in all weathers catching shrimp, his long hours only being equalled by those of the child's mother, as she steamed, peeled and packed the tiny shell fish. Having sampled the results of their efforts I can only say how superb the delicacy was and how much I appreciated their efforts.

The days hurried by and, before I knew it, the working week was drawing to a close. On the first Friday morning, Doctor Oxford kindly asked me if I should like to invite a friend up for the weekend. 'She could be accommodated in the house, there must be a room somewhere,' the doctor said. I appreciated her concern for me but never the less, I felt slightly embarrassed when I told her

'that a friend was indeed coming up to visit me and my friend was a he'

'I see,' said the doctor in a tone that implied slight disapproval. 'He will not be able to stay in the house of course,' she added a bit primly. Oh dear I thought, black mark to Betsy. I could see the good lady was a bit dismayed at the thought of a gentleman caller and I hastened to try to reassure her all was perfectly proper and arrangements had been made for my friend to stay at a hotel in Windermere. The disconcerted doctor relaxed a little at that. It had obviously reassured her, in some minor way, that she was not harbouring the harlot of the hills in her professional bosom.

Doctor Oxford did not have to spell it out. I knew the place was an enclosed order. I did not want Roland to stay there anyway, apart from the paucity of the food and the grim meal times, I was looking forward to the heady social life of Bowness or Ambleside.

Explaining she was going away for the weekend, Doctor Oxford alerted me to the fact the hospital doors were always locked promptly at ten thirty. So bidding me an enjoyable weekend she disappeared until Monday.

I had to confess I was mightily relieved to see Roland's old banger sweep up the drive early on Friday evening. What was that I had told myself a few days ago about him being so sure of me? Certainly all my indignation had vaporised with the passage of a very few days in this place. Mind you I told myself, no point in telling him how constricting life is here, though one wouldn't have to be Conan Doyle to work that out in very quick time.

I had carefully positioned myself in the drawing room when the maid announced there was a gentleman for Miss Arden. I rose quickly, I could see Roland standing in the doorway and knew he was being scrutinised by the patently curious Sisters.

I don't think I have ever been more relieved to see a boyfriend, something I am sure that Roland picked up on. Of course he didn't know at that moment he was my link to civilisation and what is more, to plentiful supplies of food. I was starving. Sure enough Roland noticed the warmth of my greeting and happily hurried me out to his waiting car before speeding away down the drive.

'What do you want to do,' he asked, once out of sight of the house. He had stopped the car and kissed me on the cheek 'and where do you want to go?'

'I think we had better head for Ambleside with all speed,' I replied. 'This place gets locked, bolted and barred at ten thirty, so I'll have to be back before then.'

We went to Ambleside and straight away into a café to get some much needed nourishment for Betsy. Afterwards we went to the cinema to see a forgettable film. In fact we left before it ended so there would be time to get some fish and chips and then enable us to be back before the ceremonial bolting of the front door. Even with hurrying, we didn't manage to beat the curfew.

'It's only a little after ten thirty,' I moaned, 'I'm too late!' The place was in complete darkness. There were no lights outside the house and certainly no light coming from inside. To cap it all, the house was too far away from the road to benefit from any scarce illumination that might have been there. I tried the handle of the front door again some what halfheartedly, it was locked of course.

'Never mind,' said Roland. 'I'll find a downstairs window, there must be one with all these rooms.'

'Be careful we don't want to frighten the children,' I whispered. We circled the house for a likely window.

'This one will do,' said Roland as he managed to push up the lower section of a small sash window. 'I think it's a pantry window you will be quite safe there, come on I'll give you a leg up.' With that he grabbed me about the knees and hoisted me aloft. A bit surprised by the vigorous way in which I was projected up, I grabbed the windowsill to do a sort of forward roll through the open window. Suddenly there was a pinging noise and I was catapulted backwards.

'What are you doing?' Asked Roland in a barely disguised whisper.

'I can't get in for some reason,' I replied.

'Try again' called Roland simultaneously yoiking my legs and the rest of me up. This time I managed to protect my face and head with one hand.

'It is no use,' I called down, 'something is preventing me. I can't see what it is but I think it might be a fly screen stopping me getting in' I let myself down to the ground again and tried to smooth down my ruffled skirt.

'This is quite fatuous and very undignified,' said Roland. Roland was one to mind about dignity and I had often teased him about it but on this occasion, I heartedly agreed with him, it was certainly ridiculous.

Without any more prevarication, Roland walked up to the front door and rang the bell. Even though I knew that Roland was right, I was not looking forward to the frosty reception that was bound to follow. On the other hand I was not going to spend the night in the flowerbed or any bed other than my own if it came to that.

After Roland had yanked the wire doorbell in a very emphatic manner we stood back and awaited events. In the blackness and quiet, the bell sounded as loud as the bells of Notre Dame. Moments later, footsteps sounded and a light switched on. The heavy door opened and a predictably disgruntled, night Sister peered round the half open door.

'Good evening,' I said with as much regality, as I could muster, 'thank you for coming to the door.' The Sister didn't say anything so much as grunt. 'Thank you, for a lovely evening Doctor Thatcher,' I deliberately announced, see you tomorrow as arranged.

'Right,' said Roland with a grin, 'I'll be round early. Good night,' he nodded to the Sister and walked away. Then, knowing all this was being duly recorded by the night staff, I closed the door softly and hurried off to my bedroom.

CHAPTER THIRTY-TWO

Roland and Food A'Plenty

The next day Saturday was totally ours. Roland called for me early and in the glorious early morning sunshine we headed for the Langdale Pikes. The weather was quite perfect. In the autumn sunshine, the sky was crystal clear, there was no dust in the atmosphere to haze the magnificent views.

Together we climbed the distinctive peaks and neighbouring areas returning to the waiting car in the early evening, tired but happy. We were as hungry as hunters and wasting the very minimum of time we changed from our thick wool socks and climbing boots into something more acceptable, ready for the swanky hotel we had earmarked for dinner.

The hotel lived up to the initial impression we had when we first saw it. It was luxuriously warm and comfortable, the hot food delicious and reassuringly plentiful. Roland and I tucked in as if there was no tomorrow which as far as I and the food and the orthopaedic hospital was concerned, there wasn't.

Later that night, we made doubly certain we were back before 'lock up.' I didn't want to run the gauntlet a second time and establish myself as 'wanton of Windermere.'

The next day Sunday was equally pleasant if not more so. Roland called for me sufficiently early to take me to Meeting in Ambleside. There is an old, established Quaker Meeting house in Ambleside and Friends' numbers are always boosted by the many tourists who visited the area all year round. We were greeted very warmly by the local folk at Meeting, who as always, could spot visitors in their midst. The Quaker Meeting closed with the handshake of two members signifying the end of the hour's silent worship. Moments later, an elderly couple came over to greet us and warmly shook hands and introduced themselves. They asked where we were from and hearing we were from Manchester and I was at the Children's hospital, kindly invited us to their home to share their lunch with them.

We declined their generous invitation as graciously as we could, explaining to our newly found friends we had booked lunch at a hotel some miles distant and that we only had an hour or so left afterwards before Roland had to return to Manchester. Nodding their understanding, the kindly couple wished us a happy day together. I felt a little mean we did not take up their offer of hospitality but on the other hand I felt it would have been ill-mannered to share someone's lunch and then dash away immediately afterwards and Roland agreed.

We drove away from Ambleside and passing though much-loved Grasmere, went on to Keswick. After a while we turned west towards Bassenthwaite Lake. We travelled along the western side of the lake until we came to a 'T' junction. Pulling into the courtyard of what at first seemed a very indifferent pub, Roland stopped the car.

'Out we get then,' he announced. I followed him, secretly a little disappointed in his selection of our lunch venue. Roland didn't say anything, just held the door open for me and I stepped inside. Once inside we passed through glass doors, well away from the public bar and immediately my doubts vanished.

We entered an elegant, sparkling clean, dining room bedecked with gleaming silver and glass wear. Immediately we were greeted by a friendly, plump, woman who showed us to our seats and straight after, a young waiter arrived with a basket full of assorted, freshly baked homemade bread rolls. Oh boy, things certainly looked promising.

The dining room was clearly a recent addition to the old building, and it had been added to very sympathetically. The lovely large windows gave magnificent views of the fells in the near distance. In the immediate foreground, there were delightful gardens, a swimming pool, and tennis courts in fact everything for everyone.

Our lunch was wonderful. From the homemade soup, to the bewildering variety of sweets, it was a gastronomic epic. I asked Roland how he had found this place and he replied he hadn't but that it had been greatly recommended by a chap at work.

After such a lunch, our zeal for strenuous exercise seemed to have vaporised, instead we decided to explore the tiny town of Cockermouth. As we strolled through the quaint town, we saw flowerbeds containing anemones in wonderful jewelled colours. I was amazed they should be growing so far north until Roland reminded me about the Gulf Stream.

The afternoon began to merge into early evening and although neither of us mentioned it, we knew that soon Roland would have to be getting back. We walked to the car in silence. The sun had gone and with it some of the carefree spirit of the day.

As we drove towards Windermere, the conversation began to regain some of its momentum. We began to discuss what we would do and where we would go on my return to the big city. It was all a bit speculative though, because I had my final examinations looming. I needed to get back into the pattern of my studies as quickly as possible. I felt as if I had been away ages and I needed the stimulus of the academic world, the lectures and my fellow students. At least my 'PhD friend,' knew all about that and understood just how keen I was to pass my finals. Still it was very pleasant to make plans, however vague.

Roland left me at the hospital door and squeezing my hand said, 'see you next weekend,' and walked quickly away. I waved as the car disappeared away down the drive. I was in time for supper and even though I'd had a wonderful lunch I knew I ought to go to the dining room for the light repast. I skipped upstairs to have a quick wash and comb my hair, there was no time to moon over Roland's departure.

I was glad to see Sister Ellis in to supper. She and Sister Jones, who only worked days, were the only ones, amongst the nursing staff, that had made me feel welcome. Both Sisters were well beyond retiring age but hugely experienced and greatly loved by the children. Sister Ellis was the relief night Sister and only worked Sunday nights. She seemed to enjoy the break from the other aspects of her personal life and of course, it gave her a sense of being needed still. She was good company and as there were only the two of us into supper, the mealtime was very pleasant indeed. When supper was over we went to the Sisters' drawing room and making ourselves comfortable, switched on the radio. We had discovered we were both fans of the 'Any Questions' series, and being the only persons in the room we were going to indulge ourselves. Freddie Grisewood was in the 'chair, it was all good stuff and my elderly companion chuckled appreciatively as she did her knitting.

The second week absolutely raced by. I had my routine now. I knew my patients and I paced myself so I wasn't quite so worn out at the end of the day. Not that it mattered much because of the lack of transport, I was house bound.

On Wednesday, Doctor Oxford asked me if I would like a lift back to Manchester on the Saturday morning. I'd had it in mind to leave after finishing work on Friday night but I had not made any definite arrangements and it seemed churlish not to accept her kind offer. The thought of travelling back home in regal comfort in her splendid car, pretty well clinched it anyway. Doctor Oxford, it seemed, was going to visit her parents in Cheshire, 'to return their impressive car and to take delivery of her own.' I couldn't help wondering what her car would be like but didn't like to enquire. However when she had added 'that she was practically going past my front door,' there was nothing more to be said other than to thank her warmly for her thought.

I was sorry to leave my small patients; the children had become my friends in the last two weeks. Apart from that though, I was secretly relieved I was to return to the bosom of my Alma Mater. The experience at Windermere had definitely taught me one thing, which was I would never actively seek employment in a small hospital, where I was to work on my own. Some people prefer to work solo but if I had learned nothing else in the last fortnight it was I would be happiest in a teaching environment.

Saturday arrived at last. I went round and said my 'goodbyes' to all the children as I promised. Some were touchingly saddened at my departure but cheered up quickly when I pointed out that as it was Saturday their parents would soon be there to see them. I shook hands with the ward Sisters, they had thawed out a bit since the first ghastly day or two or perhaps it was because I was leaving, which ever, it did not matter.

Predictably, Doctor Oxford arrived promptly. I loaded my case into the car boot then settled down next to her in the front, luxuriating in the comfortable leather upholstery. Doctor Oxford started the engine imperceptibly and silently the car pulled away from the front door and glided away down the drive. I did not look back. I would be out of sight and out of mind in minutes, I thought.

Doctor Oxford sat quietly for the first mile or so then launched pleasantly into conversation. She enquired if I had enjoyed my stay? I replied I had and that I had found the work different and interesting. It had not pushed back the frontiers of my orthopaedic experience to any great extent, I thought silently but it had taught me a valuable lesson on how to pace myself, I told the Doctor that as a student the work was allocated and therefore the pacing was done for you and you just don't realise the importance of that until you were thrown in at the deep end. The doctor smiled and briefly glanced at me, agreeing that it was an important part of the learning curve. There was also for me, privately, the invaluable lesson of responsibility when working by oneself. The job is yours alone, it is what you make of it and your patients recover or not accordingly as the case may be. What the last two weeks had really done for me however, was to make me look realistically to my future as far as my work was concerned. More than anything else, it confirmed my hitherto unrecognised suspicion I would be most happy in a large teaching establishment attached to a medical school. Before 'Windermere,' it had only been a vague feeling but this last fortnight had concentrated my thinking. I was grateful I had learned that much without having to commit myself for a much longer and possibly expensive period, of more than two weeks.

The drive back to Manchester was very pleasant; Doctor Oxford was a quiet charming woman and an extremely interesting person. When we eventually arrived at our house, she declined an invitation to join us for lunch explaining her parents were elderly and would be worried if she did not appear on time.

Thanking her for all her help and support, we said goodbye and giving me a cheery wave, she glided away in that superb sedan never to meet up again, sadly.

My family were delighted to see me back home and waited eagerly to hear about my experiences, as I put my case down and took my coat off. I told them of the horrors of the first night, the grim food, the standoffish ward Sisters and by being locked out on the Saturday night at thirty-one minutes passed ten. I told them about my little patients, how young and brave they were and my parents nodded sympathetically. I told them about the lovely people at Ambleside Meeting, we had met, some of whom my parents knew. I told them about Roland's visit and how he had saved me from near starvation with the delicious meals. I told them how very supportive Doctor Oxford had been and how she had driven me home in that super car and dropped me off but declined my invitation to lunch with us citing her anxious, aged parents waiting for her in Alderley Edge. My family laughed as I told them about trying to get into the hospital by the pantry window and Roland's exasperation at the whole situation. 'I could just imagine him,' my mother had said as she chuckled at the thought.

There certainly was no question about starvation at my mother's table and we all tucked into a delicious lunch after which I went upstairs to unpack and sleep.

That evening, as arranged in Windermere, I met Roland at the university dance. I knew just where he would be waiting for me in the building and sure enough there he was, tall, dignified and pleased to see me. We danced the night away and after driving me home, arranged to pick me up a bit later than usual, next morning. I told him I looked forward to that especially as the Indian summer seemed to be still holding out.

CHAPTER THIRTY-THREE

Called To Account

Back at the hospital on Monday morning, it was lovely to walk into Fiona first thing who, reassuringly, said she had missed me. She asked me how I got on and did I manage alright or did I have any problems that I thought I couldn't handle? Typical of Fiona, the questions came quietly and quickly. I told her I thought I managed OK, and I didn't think I had problems that I couldn't handle but perhaps Bo was going to tell me differently when I got the call to see her. 'Oh I'm certain you managed very well,' said my loyal friend comfortingly.

As nine o'clock approach more of my friends appeared and they stood in a group around me asking questions. They stared in utter disbelief as I told them about the awful meagre meals and were gratifyingly sympathetic when I told them about the ghastly nightmare of arriving the first night to be greeted by the bluebottle episode. As nine o'clock struck we hurried down the corridor, Fiona, at my side, saying, 'that it is as if you are describing a completely different place to the one we all visited in the summer,' then my learned friend added

'all that glisters,' and I nodded, how very true.

Predictably Bo sent for me that morning and wanted to know how I had got on. I told her I thought I had managed reasonably well and we talked briefly about what sort of cases I had and how I had treated them. I certainly didn't tell her about the frosty ward Sisters or the dreadful bluebottle episode, not to mention the near starvation diet. 'Maybe one day when we were qualified we would talk about such things and laugh about it,' I said to Fiona later. As I was about to leave her office Bo said that.

'Doctor Oxford had spoken highly of you and thought you managed very well. Well done Miss Arden, of course I expected nothing less.' I walked away from Bo's office, cheered and reassured, any doubts that had been lingering about my stay at Windermere, well and truly dashed, greatly to my relief.

By mid-morning, I realised two of our set were missing. Over coffee

I asked Barbara what had happened to those two. She told me they were at Monsall Isolation Hospital helping out; Sylvia and I were going next week. While I had been away, the polio epidemic, which had started in the early Summer, and was growing as I left, had escalated alarmingly, to the extent the staff at the isolation hospital were totally run off their feet and were needing help desperately. The general public knew the number of cases was increasing and they were justifiably concerned but they had no idea about the true numbers that were actually being notified to the Medical Officer of Health. The numbers were underplayed in the press, to prevent any panic. Even so, the increasing numbers in the public eye became apparent when large banners were strung across major road intersections such as Cambridge Street and Oxford Street, in Manchester, appealing for volunteers.

It was the last great outbreak of poliomyelitis in Europe and America for soon after the decline of the epidemic, the Salk vaccine, discovered in the USA, became available worldwide.

The head of the physiotherapy department at Monsall was an old girl of Bo's and it was to her that Mrs Kelly turned for help. The staff at Monsall were dropping with exhaustion. The hospital was crammed with patients with acute polio, some of whom, in fact many of whom, were in iron lungs. When the request came to Bo for any help at all, she summoned her senior students and asked them if they would like to volunteer.

As Bo asked for volunteers, she pointed out the distinct risk of catching this highly infectious disease, especially as it had a predisposition for children and young people. Not for nothing was the disease known as 'infantile paralysis.' Only students, who were over twenty-one, the then age of consent, could volunteer, Bo had said. Not surprisingly, Bo was feeling very responsible for her students who, just by reason of age, were vulnerable. As it happened, for one reason or another, none of the male students were able to volunteer. Some were married with young children, others like Fiona lived a considerable distance away and another two bus trips each way, were just two too many. Then of course there were those students who felt they should only concentrate on their finals quite understandably. Whatever one decides, as Bo had said that it must be entirely up to us to choose, I and everyone concerned, would quite understand whatever you decide.

That night, going home, I became more aware of the gravity of the situation when I took the time to read the banners that were strung across major city road intersections, asking for volunteers of all categories. The banners, asked for porters, nurses, and helpers of all description, to apply at once. This I was told later was to allow the permanent staff to have at least one day off, the first in weeks. Things were grave indeed.

As I sat on the bus going home at the end of my first day back, I couldn't help think about the changes that had taken place, seemingly overnight, especially about the frightful business of the polio epidemic. I had listened to Barbara when she said 'she and Sylvia would be going to Monsall next week for a two week stint'. Apparently because of the coming exams, two weeks was the fixed term for the volunteers. I had asked my friends whether they were concerned about catching polio?

'Well yes,' Barbara had replied, 'I suppose we are but we are getting paid and I am flat broke.'

'And,' added Sylvia, as if it explained everything, 'we will get vaccinated.' When we all knew there was no real protection then against the disease.

I stepped off the bus and walked the short distance to my home. As I opened the door my mother was there waiting for me, to find out what the feedback from Windermere was and what Bo had said. I took my coat off and sank down on a kitchen chair thankful for the steaming hot cup of tea my mother had poured. I told her all that had happened and what Bo had said and what Doctor Oxford had told Bo and how everyone seemed to think I had done a good job. I then went on to tell my mother about Bo's request for volunteers to go to Monsall. My mother sat there listening quietly as I told her the pros and cons of going there. Though, as I itemised things, I thought on the face of it there did not seem many pros, particularly bearing in mind the short time left before finals. After a while, my mother asked if I would go? I told her that I expect I would and it would be interesting to see if the place has changed much since I had spent a mandatory four weeks there as a child, suffering from scarlet fever. My mother nodded her understanding. She knew I would be very interested in the work. She would have loved the opportunity to have trained as a doctor herself, but as she had four sisters and five brothers, that was not an option. My mother's family had been reasonably well off but it was just that the girls were not expected or allowed aspirations other than those of the matrimonial type.

Regarding my proposed trip to Monsall and just to clinch the matter, I added that we would be paid too. 'Splendid,' my mother had replied 'and it would be very useful for the coming Christmas, but she wondered how your father would feel about it all?' Surprisingly, my father having listened to my debrief session with Bo later in the evening, did not give an opinion on my possible venture to Monsall. I knew he was concerned, as was my mother and the rest of my family but I also knew that, if having given it thought, and I wanted to go, then that was the right decision and they would support me whole heartedly.

CHAPTER THIRTY-FOUR

Polio Epidemic

It wasn't long before Bo sent me a summons to attend her office. I knocked and waited and as I entered thought, strange, I have lost all my nervousness these days. Not that anyone ever became familiar with the Principal, I certainly did not but somehow or other subconsciously, I had discovered she was only human after all.

'I have been speaking to Doctor Oxford again on the phone,' Bo started. 'She wished me to tell you how pleased and grateful she was for your efforts. She particularly wanted me to wish you well in your finals.'

I stood there trying to find words to express my gratitude for these kind remarks but I didn't seem to be making a very good job of it. Instead I stood there listening and nodding my appreciation.

'Of course,' Bo moved on briskly 'I told her I didn't expect any less of my students but it is nice to be told. Now about the polio epidemic.' Bo changed the subject abruptly in her characteristic manner. 'Are you interested in doing a spell at Monsall?' Bo continued without giving me time to reply. 'If you are, I suggest that you go in two-weeks' time which would give you time to do any revision you have planned, beforehand.'

'Any revision that I might have' I thought to myself, 'I haven't started yet.'

'That would give you two weeks there,' Bo continued, 'and three weeks here before the start of the finals.' It was quite clear from her conversation that Bo expected me to say yes to the proposition. 'You are quite at liberty to turn down the offer for whatever reason whatsoever.' She added, 'You must do which ever you would prefer to do, it is absolutely voluntary.'

I listened to what Bo had to say but as she had guessed I had already decided to go if asked. I had been thinking about it ever since the conversation I'd had with Barbara, on my first day back after Windermere. I had made up my mind to get some experience on the acute polio unit if invited to do so. I told Bo my thoughts on the matter.

'I think you are very wise to go' she replied. 'Polio along with other killer diseases will soon be conquered or at least controlled with developing vaccines. But,' she continued, 'it is a worldwide disease and in a rather sad way we, as physiotherapists here, now, have a unique opportunity to gain this valuable experience.' As she spoke it was as though she was thinking out loud rather than speaking to me. 'In the coming years most medical staff will not see polio, tetanus, diphtheria or even tuberculosis and possibly have difficulty in recognising it, when and if, it presents itself.'

As soon as I left Bo's office, I went to the medical library. There were several publications on the pathology of polio but very little on the actual treatment of the disease. Collecting a variety of books about me, I found a quiet corner and began to read. It was an incredibly interesting subject in its pathology, with its sudden onset and affinity for children and young people. As I placed the book I was reading down, I saw a small publication slip out of the book, it was headed, *Hot Pack Treatment for Infantile Paralysis.* As I turned the pages I vaguely remembered there was some controversy, many years before about the 'hot-pack treatment,' which was advocated by an Australian woman, Sister Kenny. The hot packs were applied to the painful muscles and joints, they were easy to heat, easy to apply and easy to move around. The treatment seemed very sensible on the face of it and I wondered what the controversy was about, considering that the only treatment then was, bed rest

Apparently the treatment was controversial because Sister Kenny was advocating, hot packs, even in the highly febrile stage. When temperatures were high, the opponents had said hot packs were contra indicated, which did seem logical. However, I thought, hot packs don't have to be hot, they obviously aren't hot enough to burn in any case but you could use warm packs to relieve the pain. Anybody who has had a bad dose of the flu knows how comforting a hot water bottle is to aching limbs, even when you have a temperature. I was beginning to think Sister Kenny's problem might have been in the word *hot* when warm might have been what she meant. I had not realised until then just how incredibly painful acute polio was but clearly I was soon to find out. In the latter stages, I continued to read, all that was offered were splints and walking aids. The polio victims were very much on their own after the first few weeks, it seemed.

Gathering up the books I wanted, I signed for them and went back to the department in considerable thought. I couldn't wait to get to Monsall.

Meanwhile Barbara and Sylvia had gone to do their stint on the polio unit and Paula and Meg had returned. They seemed to have found the work interesting and were delighted to be paid, particularly in cash. It had been hard work they said and at first a bit scary but they soon got into the routine. The work was heavy, a lot of lifting and of course because it was an isolation hospital, the wards all stood independently in the grounds. Unfortunately for Meg and Paula the weather had been wet the whole of their two weeks and they spent a great deal of time running between the units, dodging the downpours, trying not to get drenched. By and large they were glad to be back at Salford and in the relative dry, although as Paula said, 'the wages did come in mighty handy.'

CHAPTER THIRTY-FIVE

Full Circle

While waiting for my time to go to Monsall Isolation Hospital I joined some of our set on the way to the medical gym across the quad. The rest of the term was to be devoted to practical sessions using the first-year students as patients and the lectures to be, of the recap variety. As one of the lecturers had pointed out it was too late in the day to be teaching you how to be physiotherapists, the aim of these lectures is to polish up your examination technique.

There was always wild speculation as to what conditions the examiners would ask us about, ranging from the totally unheard of, to the ridiculously common place and therefore often overlooked, simple, everyday complaints.

On our way, passing through another department, I could see some junior students practising setting up various apparatus under the watchful eye of a male lecturer. There were several groups of students dotted about in small work clusters. One group was standing by a plinth trying to assemble the traction apparatus for treating the lumbar spine. The poor student was sitting on a stool with a tense look on her face as her colleagues applied the leather straps under her chin and around the back of her head, which looked more like the bridle for a horse than anything remotely therapeutic. Another set of straps was securely tightened around the student's hips and the whole thing connected to a special clock face that measured the pull of the traction in pounds weight. It was fairly obvious to those of us just passing by, that the poor girl, who was being subjected to her colleagues therapy, felt that she had a great deal in common with torture chambers and mediaeval prisoners in days of yore.

Suddenly there was a bellow from another corner of the department. We all turned our heads as one man. There a poor girl was trying desperately to adjust the neck traction, on a fellow student. She had assembled the equipment wrongly and almost lethally.

'Miss Ward!' Shouted the exasperated male lecturer, rapidly going to the rescue of the 'patient,' 'perhaps I should call you Pierpoint, the onetime State executioner. Miss Ward,' he continued, 'at this hospital, the effect of treatment is supposed to be the relief of pain, not the final solution, and we would like to maintain that tradition.'

The student who was supposed to be treating her 'patient' blushed a bright red but it did not compare with the cyanosed complexion of her brave but up until then, choking friend. The poor girl, who was the acting patient, would have fallen over had she not been sitting on a stool. Her torso was being held upright by the head traction gear, which had slipped around her neck, almost disastrously.

'Good god!' Muttered Sylvia, as we all stood and looked at the near catastrophe in horror, 'I think we had better move on fast.'

As we entered the medical gym we saw our 'models' sitting on the low gym benches awaiting our arrival. Also waiting was Bo, her toe tapping, as she saw us sauntering in.

'Come on, get a move on,' Bo announced briskly, 'there is work to be done!'

We were each allocated a junior student. The first year students were always the victims for two reasons. Firstly they were the most readily spared from other work, supposing that they had actually been lucky enough to have had any contact with a real patient by now. Secondly, because they were new students, they were presumably ignorant and therefore not able to assist their senior colleagues who might be in exam difficulties.

The first year students were told to strip to bra and pants. I could see the embarrassed looks on their faces as they did so. My mind went back to three years ago when we too, were in exactly the same position and how awkward we had felt and I sympathised. Some of the students were in their underwear but some poor souls were wearing less depending on which bit of their anatomy was under scrutiny.

As usual, Fiona and I paired off and being allocated a student began our work. We were told by Bo we should firstly mark out both the arterial and venous blood vessels and the cervical and brachial plexus of the arm and upper trunk, having first made note of any deformities or unusual features that our patient might have. The student wasn't deformed in any way of course, other than having her right shoulder somewhat elevated, probably due to carrying her school bags on her right shoulder for years, easily correctable once it was pointed out to the girl. She also stood 'in toed' a bit which we pointed out and which she also corrected at once, standing with her feet directly forward and parallel. Bo came over to watch us in action.

'This is a middle aged woman who has just had a total pneumonectomy, forty eight hours ago,' she said, stopping us. 'What are your aims of treatment and how would you treat her?'

Thankfully both of us had done a brief stint at Baguley Sanatorium in Wythenshawe, when we worked on the post-op ward, so having had a patient that had a lung removed was not totally new to us. We discussed with Bo about the absolute need to keep the remaining lung aerated and to prevent secretions gathering. This meant teaching the patient to cough while we, gently but firmly, supported the operation site on the front and back of the chest wall simultaneously. It isn't easy for the patient who is in considerable post op discomfort, frightened and understandably very reluctant to cough. At Baguley the patients were given little sips of neat-fresh lemon juice in warm water, which seemed to help them to cough. Posture was also important. It was essential the patient did not collapse down on the side where the lung had been removed, very easy to do by the patient as they, almost by reflex, protected their sore side. All these things we discussed with Bo who looked reasonably satisfied with our answers.

I was given a 'new model.' She had been sitting on the gym bench waiting to be called. The girl who was to be my model was painfully embarrassed and I felt for her.

'Just stand naturally, feet apart a little and look straight ahead,' I said. A bit ridiculous I thought to myself, who stands 'quite naturally' in this situation; still we have to go through the routine. I examined the model and asked her if she thought that she was standing correctly?

'Er yes I think so,' came the tentative reply. To illustrate what I was getting at, I wheeled the portable long length mirror over and asked her to stand in front of it and look at herself. As soon as she glimpsed her reflection she instinctively adjusted her stance. We all do it. Even so she did seem to check whether her abdominal muscles were tucked and were her legs best displayed. When I asked her whether her eyes, ears and shoulders were level and parallel she took a new critical look at herself and adjusted her stance, checking without being told that her chin should be over her sternum.

'Good for you,' I had said and she smiled in appreciation and relaxed a bit. While she was trying to correct all the slight oddities that we all develop, I went to examine her back. I was scribbling furiously in case Bo came back, some lack of symmetry is normal. It is the ability to recognise the permissible irregularity from the pathological unacceptable that separates the truly skilled from the apparently skilled.

Having checked the visible I now had to check the not so visible. All joint movements had to be gone through systematically. As I was checking the range of movement in my model's shoulder joint, I caught a glimpse of Fiona who had been given a male first year student for her next model. Fiona and he were in a small room off ours, the door was ajar and I recognised the student. He was very keen on weight lifting and bodybuilding and although not too tall was very muscular. Fiona was trying to obtain a greater range of shoulder movement than her model was apparently offering. Fiona was urging him to put his fingers on his shoulders but because he had bulging biceps, triceps and deltoids, he couldn't get anywhere near his shoulders with his finger tips. I heard Fiona urging him, 'to tuck your elbows into your waist, now, touch your shoulders.' In normally built people this is easily done but not so in that male student. He tried to oblige but his bulky triceps held his upper arms away from his body and his bulging biceps held his fingers well away from his shoulders. Fiona gave up and moved on.

At last the session was over, the grinning models looking like something out of an old Red Indian movie with their major arteries marked in red, veins in blue and major nerves in yellow, just as we had been years ago. I collected my bag and moved over to my friends who were standing in a group near the door.

'Did you see my model?' Exclaimed Fiona. 'He is absolutely muscle bound.'

'Yes I could see you were having a few problems there' and laughed as she pulled a face.

CHAPTER THIRTY-SIX

Christmas 1941: Blitz

At last the Monday morning arrived when it was my turn to present myself at Monsall, or the fever hospital as the local citizens called Monsall. There were the fever vans, the green ambulances, in their own special livery, denoting to everyone that they only carried patients with infectious diseases and were therefore feared, as opposed to the maroon ambulances that carried all other patients, whatever they were suffering from.

I had taken the bus to the centre of Manchester as usual and crossed Piccadilly gardens to Stevenson Square. At one time, before the days of the welfare state, it was in Stevenson's Square that the poor and destitute would gather at night. Collecting wood and any other combustible material, from the local markets, they would make themselves a bonfire to keep themselves warm, the police moving them on before dawn. No sign of that now I thought as I saw my bus standing there at its terminus. I hopped on the bus, joining a few other people just before it moved off and sat down watching the unfamiliar part of Manchester unfold itself.

The bus conductor suddenly called out 'Monsall Hospital,' I hurried along the bus and jumped off just in time. There it was, a sombre edifice with a high wall round the grounds, which ended in a massive set of wrought iron gates. As I approached the gates they were open, indicating too much traffic passing through all the time, to bother closing them especially in daytime.

I entered through the gateway, walked past the porter's lodge and as instructed, headed for the physiotherapy department to find the head of department, Miss Kelly.

'Hello,' said Miss Kelly as I entered the department. 'I'm Ann Kelly,' coming to meet me with her arm outstretched, ready to shake mine. 'Thanks for volunteering to help out.' Ann was a pleasantly built woman in her mid-thirties I guessed. As she greeted me in a somewhat breathless way, I thought that she must have been hurrying. It did not take long to discover that this apparent breathlessness, was a speech characteristic of hers. She spoke like that, as a matter of habit, indicating haste or an emergency, real or apparent, but her friendly cheerfulness, put one at ease straight away.

'Come along,' she panted when she had shown me where to put my coat. 'You have to have some jabs before you go on the wards.' Then, not very reassuringly she said, 'Of course it would have been much better if you'd had them a few days ago and then you would have been protected before you start, but it's a bit late now.' Yes, I thought but here goes.

We entered the medical Director's office and Ann introduced me. A moment later I was face down being injected with two huge doses of gamma globulin, one into each side of my bottom. This was immediately before the Salk vaccine became available. Gamma globulin apparently stimulated one's own natural antibodies, hopefully fighting off any of the lurking viruses that might have the temerity to attack me.

'Well, that's that,' said the cheerful doctor before adding, 'you will feel like you have been kicked by a mule for the next three or four days and you will walk as if you have been too, but it will wear off.' Great I thought I shall no doubt, be the belle of the ball tomorrow night. I wonder what Roland will say when I try a stiff legged foxtrot. I had not mentioned to him I was about to go to Monsall.

Doctor Patterson was a charming man who was undoubtedly pleased to see extra help arriving and said as much. As he walked with us, I had the pleasurable feeling that I, and the rest of Bo's volunteers, were a cross between the U.S. Cavalry and Angels of Mercy.

'Arrangements have been made for you to collect your pay at the office and you should know by now what hours you will be working,' said the paternal Patterson

I nodded.

'Good,' he said, 'I will see you about the hospital, I hope you won't be too stiff tonight.' Smiling my thanks at the kindly doctor, I followed Ann thinking that if I am not careful I could feel martyred to the cause with all this gratitude.

'I will show you the lay out of the wards first of all,' Ann began, in her quiet breathless manner. 'At the moment there are two main categories, the acute and the post-acute, nobody stays here after that stage, at the moment, there just isn't room nor the staff.'

As we walked through the grounds, I tried to see if there was anywhere that seemed familiar. Many years before as a toddler, I had to spend a whole month here at Monsall. I didn't recognise the ward only the fact that in common with all isolation hospitals and sanatoria, the units were built as separate entities in the large grounds. Purposely there were no linking corridors to these far flung wards, in an attempt to contain contagion. During the long winter months one was nearly blown away or drenched in freezing rain as we commuted from ward to ward. We must have looked like something from a Lowry painting as we scurried through the grounds with our cloaks pulled tightly around us, heads down, to prevent the wind blowing off the hoods of our cloaks. The cold outside always made us gasp after the warmth of the wards inside.

My mind went back to the day my elder brother was diagnosed with scarlet fever. He was seriously ill. The doctor had been called and she announced my brother would have to go to hospital straight away for the mandatory four weeks and 'yes it had to be to Monsall.' I can still hear the dismay in my mother's voice as she heard the news and he would be away for the whole of Christmas. The thought that my brother would be alone in hospital at Christmas was too much for me so when nobody was looking I deliberately sat down on his bed hoping to get infected. I thought if I had to go into hospital too he would not be on his own at Christmas. I was wrong of course.

Later that night, the green fever van arrived, my mother was thankful it was dark and that none of the neighbours could see and treat us like lepers. Not only was it dark when my brother was loaded into the ambulance, there was no moon, it was pitch black in the enforced war-time black out, there being no street lighting and it was mid-winter. Trying to pick its way through the blacked out, fifteen miles to the hospital, the ambulance hit a cyclist. There they were, an ambulance at the scene unable to help, the 'fever van,' unable to pick up casualties. They just had to wait until the right ambulance came. I don't think the chap was badly hurt though as a small child nobody thought it necessary to inform me of such interesting details.

Alas for my poor mother within a week, I too was being bungled into the green fever van. It was mid-morning and certainly most neighbours' curtains were twitching. Somehow I had gone off the noble idea of joining my brother and clung to my mother and to her beautiful hair. One of my mother's glorious long plaits, which she wore wound in a bun on the nape of her neck had tumbled down. Her hair usually did in hectic moments regardless of the huge number of substantial hairpins involved. As a toddler I loved the smell and touch of my mother's long silky hair, it was a comfort to me and I wasn't about to let go. The nurse sent to accompany me, was getting decidedly exasperated and in an effort to break the deadlock my mother said in a falsely bright tone, 'Father Christmas is giving you a Rupert book.' I looked at the book, it did not compare to my mother and, the wartime book had no pictures.

This isn't a proper Rupert book I thought as I stubbornly held on to my mother. Of course being so small, I had no idea of how much time and effort, my parents had spent searching for the 'proper' Rupert book published by the *Daily Mail.* I had always received that colourful book at Christmas but because of the war it was just not available.

By this time the nurse had decided enough time had been wasted and took a firm line. Picking me up, she tightly wrapped both myself, and my Christmas book, in the thick, green, scratchy, hospital blanket, and ordered the driver to take me to the ambulance at once.

Lying there, in the ambulance, with the blanket wrapped so tightly about me that I was convinced I would die of suffocation long before I died of scarlet fever, the ambulance driver strapped me in. He closed the van doors and in the 'restful green' interior of the fever van, there I was, left by myself, feeling very miserable. The prim, starchy, nurse chose to ride with the driver. I felt and was very alone.

There our family was then, a week before Christmas, two children in hospital and my parents wondering if their third child, a baby, would also succumb. What was certain was my poor mother had to endure the indignity of having to have her home officially fumigated by the Council, for a second time in ten days. Apparently a chap came from the Department of Health and sprayed each room to disinfect the house of contagion.

I was still in the scratchy blanket as the ambulance driver carried me to the ward followed by the attendant nurse. We entered the women's ward at a brisk clip, all eyes were on us, as the procession marched to the very last bed, mine.

Having just had my injections of gamma globulin ready to begin work at Monsall, I couldn't help remember the seemingly excessive number of daily injections I had to have then. Being the obstinate child that I was, I was determined not to cry and I didn't but sometimes it was a close call. One day, when the nurse giving me the latest injection said, 'well at least you don't cry,' it occurred to me that perhaps I ought to wail and perhaps they would stop.

My stay in hospital was purely routine. I was not really ill unlike my brother who was. We were in hospital during the great blitz on Manchester. During this time, Manchester was to endure the worst and most prolonged blitz on the city as the bombers sought out the great engineering conglomerates, the docks, mines and the textile mills, all of which were sustaining Britain. For two days and nights Manchester was attacked incessantly with hundreds of incendiary bombs lighting up the city for the following bombers.

All the patients had been moved onto the floor, on their mattresses, under the beds. Because I was so young, I was not frightened but rather enjoyed what

I thought was the giant firework display outside, as the incendiaries rained down on the hospital. I was also intrigued by the unusual, busy bustle that was going on in the ward. Now and again there were huge flashes outside that lit up the ward as if it were daylight. As I lay there watching this interesting display, a nurse hurried down the ward, picked me up and thrust me under a bed into the arms of a middle aged woman. 'There you are you won't be frightened now,' the nurse had said hurrying off in the sickening way that adults have before I could say I wasn't frightened. If I wasn't frightened, the woman that I had been put with most certainly was. She was in a blind panic.

'Here,' the woman had said, 'hold this tightly it will keep you safe,' On saying that she thrust a photograph into my hands. I had never met a hysterical adult before but I can still remember the cool distaste I felt, holding a photograph as instructed, whilst being clutched frantically in the arms of that panicking woman.

'Hold on to the photograph,' she kept urging, 'and nothing will happen to you.'

It was a blinding moment of truth for me, a moment of disillusionment. Adults were not perfect! I kept tight hold of the photograph to please the stranger I had been placed with, realising at the same time that scarlet fever was not the only thing that was infectious, fear was too.

Next morning I stood on my bed and peered out of the window, the grounds were pockmarked. The ruined, blackened, pitted lawns were smoking where the incendiaries had fallen, with firemen still trying to douse them. Word had it that all male patients who were deemed fit enough, were asked to volunteer in the night, having to get dressed and turn out to help put out the numerous incendiary fires that were endangering the hospital. My brother was one of the patients who helped and it cost him dear. He caught a further infection and had to stay in hospital another two weeks

At the same time, my father, who, after a long and tiring day at work, had to do his stint of 'fire watching,' over night, in the city centre. My father's place of business was in the old area in Manchester, near the Cathedral, where the Romans were once based and which now thanks to the prolonged bombing, had suffered badly. It was the centre of the gem and jewellery business and my father later told of his unique experience of searching for gemstones in the rubble, but of course not to keep.

As I continued towards the isolation unit, I couldn't help smile remembering my last hours here, at this hospital, as a child.

One morning lying in bed, a nurse came up to me and told me 'that I could go home later that day if my tests proved I was well enough.' She carried with her an enormous test tube sort of jar with a flat base, which she stood there in the sluice room. It threatened me by its sheer size. My job the nurse had informed me was to use the enamelled bedpan which she had placed on the sluice room floor and to give her a specimen. Now in common with many small children, try as might, I could not perform on command. Five minutes later I heard the brisk footsteps of the nurse and knew she would not be pleased.

'Keep trying, you do want to go home don't you?' She commanded.

I nodded dismally.

A good few minutes later the ward Sister came to my rescue quite unwittingly. She was bringing Beryl to the sluice on a similar mission. Now Beryl was a good five years older than me. She was a plump nine-year-old and when Sister said she would be back in a few minutes and left us to it, Beryl performed admirably. She generously poured half the contents of her bedpan into my specimen jar, saving the rest for her container. A few minutes later the first nurse could be heard marching briskly down the ward towards us.

'Good girls,' the nurse said, as she saw the results of both of our apparent efforts, 'that wasn't too difficult was it?' She continued before sending us back to our beds.

I have always been eternally grateful to Beryl not just for helping me out but more importantly, for her being fit and well. If Beryl's specimen had 'failed the lab test,' I would have had to stay in hospital, doubtless being dosed with various medications, that I didn't need for ailments from which I was not suffering.

CHAPTER THIRTY-SEVEN

Iron Lungs

Ann Kelly pushed open the doors of the Isolation Unit, and we entered a wide lobby off which sprang two diverging corridors.

'Before we go any further,' said Ann, 'we must gown up, all of the patients are barrier nursed'

In the lobby there were shelves stacked with freshly laundered linen of every description. Nearest the external doors there were piles of clean white gowns and in a nearby box, face masks. We hung up our outside clothes and put on the voluminous gowns, which went around me twice and I tied it at the waist.

'It's one size fits all,' said Ann seeing me cope with the excess material. 'It's easier that way.' She reached into the box and took two face masks, one of which she handed to me. 'When we leave this ward we must take off our gowns and masks and leave them in the wicker laundry basket over there.' I saw where she pointed and nodded.

We turned left down one of the two corridors and into a large old, fashioned ward. Inside the ward was a very peculiar sight, standing on trestles, apparently randomly placed were long, black coffin shaped boxes. The boxes were off set, with a mirror at the head. At the other end, next to the box, was a large circular tub with concertina type walls. The tub, a yard in diameter was attached to the foot of the box by way of a very large flexible hose. The tubs looked a little like enormous Chinese lanterns but they were bellows and they were attached to not coffins, but to iron lungs.

Ann and I walked over to one of the iron lungs and then I saw a head at the top end, with large eyes that had been watching us from the moment we had entered the ward, by way of the specially tilted mirror.

'Hello Jean, how are you feeling today?' Said Ann with a smile. 'This is Miss Arden, a new physio, who has come to help out and will be treating you.'

'Hello Jean,' I said.

'Hello,' whispered Jean, looking at me through her mirror.

Ann showed me how the powerful rubber flanges around her neck and inside the portholes down the side of the lung kept the lung airtight. The pumping bellows, were continually hissing as they exerted a negative pressure on the patients lungs forcing the patient's own lungs to expand by drawing in air then as the bellows fell, the patient breathed out. The portholes down the side of the lung could be opened safely to allow the patient to be treated, the nurse or physio being able to reach the patient through the thick airtight rubber seals.

It was not what I expected at all. The truth was I had no idea what to expect. But this huge room, filled with higgledy-piggledy spaced coffin-like iron lungs, plus the added noise of the many hissing, thrumming bellows, seemed like a nightmare made real. Ann sensed my feelings and without waiting to be asked she said the iron lungs were arranged so that the patients could see what was going on in the ward as much as possible. When I looked around, I could see what she meant. Each patient had their own mirror tilted and angled just above their face. Through these mirrors the patients could see most of the ward, particularly the doorway. For the first time I suddenly became aware I was being scrutinised by a dozen or so pairs of eyes.

'Here is Miss Arden everyone, a new physio' Ann called out as I looked around the room.

'Hello,' I called and waved to everybody. Those patients that could, had said hello in return, those who couldn't, just bravely smiled their welcome. Gosh, what a tragedy, I thought, all these young people in such a hideous situation.

I asked Ann 'what the couple of empty hospital beds near the door were for?' She replied that, it was a matter of urgency, critically ill patients were directly brought into this ward and the doctor would examine them to see what treatment would be best for the individual. If they couldn't breathe on their own because their intercostals muscles were paralysed they were to be transferred to a lung immediately. If they were lucky and they could breathe independently, then they were kept here under observation for a few hours just to make sure. I nodded, showing I fully understood the gravity of the situation.

As Ann introduced me to the patients in the iron lungs, I noticed that not one was over forty or younger than fifteen. Relatively speaking there were few children to adults that ended up in iron lungs. It seemed if the children were that badly affected they didn't survive, despite the best efforts of the staff.

We went round to all the patients having a quiet word with them. They all had difficulty in speaking, even the stronger patients, because they had to time their words with the rhythm of the vacuum effect of the ventilating pump. The negative pressure in the iron lungs forced the ribs to lift like a bucket handles, increasing the space capacity in the thorax, which in turn, sucked air in through the mouth. As the pressure dropped so the chest wall collapsed and the patient breathed out and they could speak albeit in a jerky manner. The pressures exerted, were carefully measured, it was obvious that a slender woman did not need as much pressure, as a well built man. Another variant was that some patients were recovering somewhat, so gradually and with the utmost caution, the pressure was reduced to encourage the patients to regain their respiratory independence. While we were talking to the patients I could see that some of the lungs were tilted down at the foot end where some were slightly tilted down at the head end all being adjusted to the respiratory needs of the individual.

Almost without exception, the history of the onset of the polio was the same, whoever I talked to. The patients would tell me how they had felt a bit poorly at first, as if they might have been getting a cold or the flu. Most of them went on to say they felt their bones aching and had a bit of muscular stiffness. Because the victims were young adults, possibly athletic men or busy young mothers, they would often try to work off their chill. This was the worst thing they could have done, for trying to work off polio, usually ended with dire results and almost certainly in permanent, paralytic damage to those muscles the sufferers were trying to 'loosen up.' Many patients told how me how they had tried to ignore what they thought was a 'touch of the flu,' only to suddenly collapse hours later.

The onset was incredibly sudden. Children might be playing in the park or have gone swimming only to find that within hours they were desperately ill, it was totally terrifying. The local authorities closed all swimming pools in an effort to control the outbreak.

The worst cases were the patients whose intercostal muscles, the muscles between the ribs, were suddenly affected. Without immediate and accurate diagnosis they were in danger of suffocation and those people, were typical of those patients in this ward.

Pushing open the ward doors, Ann and I left the ward and shedding our gowns and masks we threw them into the laundry basket where they would be taken to the hospitals own laundry to be first washed and then sterilised. We washed our hands before putting on new clean masks and gowns and headed down the opposite corridor.

CHAPTER THIRTY-EIGHT

Back Breaking

Attired in our fresh gowns, we walked down the corridor to the ward on the right hand side and entered. Here, the patients were in standard hospital beds, both men and women. These patients too, were in the acute stage of polio, to varying degrees, with high temperatures, muscle stiffness and the inevitable pain. The pain wasn't the sort we all get when we sit awkwardly for any length of time then try to move, but great pain, that is even more excruciating on touch. Unfortunately the patients did have to be touched to be nursed or to be treated by us, the physios.

'In no way was the patient to move their affected limbs on their own that would only exacerbate the situation,' said Ann. So it was our work to gently support the limbs and very cautiously put them through a full range of passive movements. That meant the physio doing all the movements to ensure the various joints did not 'gum up' and become 'frozen.' In no way, was the patient to do their own exercises in the highly febrile stage, I kept hearing Ann warn. The difficulties soon became apparent. If the patient had one group of muscles paralysed, say for example, the quadriceps at the front of the thigh, it was possible that the hamstrings at the back of the thigh were not affected. This resulted in the muscles with normal tone exerting an excessive pull on the flaccid, paralysed muscles, causing great pain and if not prevented, deformity. 'Resting,' splints, soft and well padded, were the answer. We made splints for feet, legs, wrists, arms and whatever else needing supporting. These splints had to be removed when we treated the patients and replaced when we had finished which all took a great deal of time.

Ann had continued to explain all this as we walked along and I hoped I would remember all the vital information that was coming at me, thick and fast. I fervently hoped that when I had to treat these courageous folk, I did not damage my patients more than the wretched polio virus was doing. I was grateful when she said emphatically that no weight-bearing exercises, of any type, should be done before I had first checked with her.

'Look there's Kate' Ann said as we saw another physio treating a young boy. 'She's treating Barry. I'll introduce you to her.' Ann and I went up to the physio where she introduced me to both Kate and Barry.

"Hello Barry, how are you feeling this morning?' Ann asked in a cheerful voice.

'I think I'm a little better but I still have a lot of pain' Barry replied softly.

The three of us nodded our heads in sympathy.

'I won't be long if you are waiting to start the baths,' said Kate. 'I'll meet you over at John's bed in a few minutes.'

'Right,' replied Ann, as we moved off, with me close alongside looking at her questioningly.

'As soon as the patients' temperatures are anything like normal,' she continued, 'we bathe the patients in warm water. Its primary purpose is to relieve their pain enabling us to do gentle exercises when they are supported in the water but of course we can give them a wash too, it all helps, you'll soon get the hang of things. Right now it is down to muscle power – ours!'

'This is John,' Ann said as we walked over to another young man, 'He got polio just over ten days ago. Initially he was in an iron lung but as you can see he doesn't need that now and so he was moved into this ward.'

'Hello,' I greeted John.

'But he does still have a great deal of pain,' Ann continued, while we waited for Kate to join us. 'It is right arm and both legs isn't John?'

John nodded.

'Today we were going to give you a bath,' Ann said to him 'and that will help!'

Kate joined us, wheeling a theatre trolley. John looked very apprehensive as we carefully lifted him onto the trolley and wheeled him to the bathroom. Any touch, any movement, was still acutely painful and we lifted him with the utmost care.

The bathroom was white tiled throughout with the exception of a band of bottle green tiles half way up the walls. Standing in the middle of the room was a huge white, enamelled, iron bath and under the screened off window, a large radiator giving out tropical amounts of heat. We filled the enormous bath two thirds full, with pleasantly warm water. The three of us gently lifted John, who was even more apprehensive, and slowly lowered him into the water. With Kate and Ann on either side and myself supporting his head, neck and shoulders, no matter how careful we were, we couldn't help hurting him and he cried out in pain. As John entered the soothing, supporting, warm water his expression said it all. The relief from his muscular and joint pain was almost instantaneous.

For the first time since the onset of his polio John was almost completely pain free. He relaxed while we hung over the bath supporting him. It was back breaking. As John relaxed in the buoyancy of the deep warm water and the pain disappeared, we could begin gentle limb movements. Finally, we sponged him down, and lifted him out of the tub onto the trolley where warm towels were placed ready to dry him and we took him back to his bed.

By the end of the day all the patients who were non-febrile, with no temperature, were treated in this way. The work was totally exhausting and backbreaking. As tired as we were, it was worth it. The relief of the pain for the patients was immediate and the relief lasted several hours, not surprisingly, they were understandably very grateful for that.

Ideally, I suppose these patients should have had the warm bath treatment both morning and evening but that was a physical impossibility. The whole treatment was so time consuming, nothing could be rushed and the whole of Ann's team, of four permanent physiotherapists, plus myself and one other volunteer from another teaching hospital, were run off our feet.

It was no wonder Ann had asked Bo for help, a few more weeks of this and lumbar discs would be popping for certain. The great wonder was why Ann had not asked for help sooner. I certainly understood the appeal for help I had seen on the banner fixed to the railway bridge on Oxford Street. Right now what was needed was simply more muscle power.

Apart from helping with the bathing, on my first day, I was given three patients to treat who had normal temperatures for the last twenty-four hours and were to start simple, active bed exercises. Ann reminded me I should just go gently and everything would be OK.

What I hadn't mentioned to Ann on my first day at Monsall, was I was going to a ball the next night. As the doctor who had given me my huge jabs had correctly warned, I did feel as 'if I had been kicked by a mule' and I was certainly walking as if I had. The next day, everyone in the small department laughed as we had a quick cup of coffee and I told them about my date for the coming evening.

'You will be a sight for sore eyes,' chuckled Ann, 'waltzing stiff-legged around the dance floor and you haven't told Roland yet?'

Ann let me go a few minutes early on my second day so that I could 'get into my glad rags,' as she put it, wishing me a great time that evening. I hobbled out of the gates and caught the two buses home.

My mother had a welcome cup of tea ready for me as I took off my coat.

She was eager to hear all about my day at the hospital and whether there had been any more confirmed cases admitted? I told her two more confirmed cases had been admitted and another suspected case of polio had come in but at the time of my leaving the hospital it hadn't been confirmed. My mother nodded and said what we all thought, the epidemic seemed to be easing off but was still active.

Finishing my cup of tea I went upstairs to wash and get into my dressing gown. My mother was making me a light meal prior to me getting into my lovely ball gown. I had told her after my first day at Monsall, that the food there was terrible. Today's lunch had been no better, two small sardines on a thin round of toast was dished up for our midday meal. We stared at our lunch, as it was placed before us, in total disbelief. 'Goodness' I said, I only hoped the cost of our meagre meals was subsidising the patients' food and they were doing a whole lot better than we were.' My colleagues had agreed.

Finally I was ready, arrayed in my lovely ball gown, I felt refreshed and looking forward to the evening. Roland arrived on time and we left in his 'velocipede,' as my father called his ancient car. We were early of course, well actually on time, but the 'dance shy,' would not be arriving until there was a crowd already on the ballroom floor and that suited Roland just fine.

We sat for a while catching up on the day's activities Roland telling me about the guys at work but not about his work, not that I would have understood too much about the atomic energy business anyway. Finally he asked me how my day has been. Well it was confession time. I told him about volunteering to go to Monsall to work on the polio unit and how yesterday had been my first day there, I told him about having to have two mega injections which were leaving me a little stiff in the legs but I added I was looking forward to dancing it off. Roland sat there and listened intently.

'What about me?' He suddenly asked.

'What about you?' I asked, not understanding.

'Well I might catch polio from you!'

The truth was, I hadn't given much thought to my contacts and them being at risk through my work. My family had never expressed any concern either, trusting in my judgement. I told him about the great care we took when entering and leaving the acute wards and anyway, I added indignantly that he was more likely to catch something in a crowded ballroom than he was from me. So much for my brave Sir Galahad I thought. Roland had the grace to laugh and said 'we should dance before the place filled up.' As I had worked all day with the predicted stiffness in my muscles, I was not going to let it spoil our evening. Roland, being the master dancer he was, took me in a firm hold and swept me across the dance floor, we seemed to cover every corner of the empty space. As the evening went on, the ballroom began to fill, kerbing Roland's exuberance. When Roland had his dancing lessons, I don't think he had progressed to jiving, advanced or otherwise probably by choice, because he was a traditionalist though he did his reluctant best when the place filled up, there wasn't room to do anything else.

About midnight when it became so packed that one could hardly move, Roland had said we should call it a day. I was glad. I was shattered but didn't want to be the person to say so. We walked hand in hand to his car standing there in the quad. It had been a lovely, special evening and I told Roland so and gathering me up he gave me a long kiss. We climbed into the ancient car and headed for my home. Walking me to the door, we arranged to meet up as usual at the weekend and kissing me good night, he left.

CHAPTER THIRTY-NINE

Close Call

The hard, but incredibly interesting, work at Monsall continued, bathing, exercising, making splints and treating the patients in the iron lungs. In no time at all, it was the middle of my second week when a never to be forgotten incident happened.

One of my patients was Jean, the patient in an iron lung, whom I had met on my first day. Jean was about twenty-eight-years old and a teacher by profession, still in the lung and unable to move any of her limbs when an emergency occurred that nearly frightened her to death and didn't do much for my heart either.

Jean was married and had one child a little girl, five-years old. She was, she told me, her eyes shining at the thought, very happily married. As I was treating her through the portholes, she would tell me about her life and how at the end of each day, she would curl up in bed next to her husband and secretly think how very lucky she was. She was an intelligent woman who had already been in her lung more than three weeks. She had seen other people come and go and she was now realising that she might be seriously and permanently paralysed. 'It was definitely on the cards' as she put it.

My patient was making some improvement though. At first she could not breathe independently at all if her iron lung was switched off even momentarily. Just in case of an emergency there were always two independent electricity supplies, one from the mains and one other an auxiliary supply in case of mains power failure.

However, gradually Jean was building up a degree of independent breathing on her own. She had learnt that by using her neck and shoulder muscles to assist her feeble intercostals lift her chest wall, she could breath at least for a short time. It meant the utmost careful supervision by the physiotherapist and I would stand very close to her head, with a stop watch in hand, as the pump was switched off for maybe no more than five seconds at first. Jean could breathe by herself longer than that of course, before we tried switching off the pump, but you had to factor in panic by the patient and who would not feel like panicking in such circumstances. It is utterly impossible to imagine how truly frightening it is to lie flat, sealed in an iron lung, I know, I tried it on my third day and I could breathe on my own. The feeling of utter helplessness and dependency on the operator who is about to switch off your life support requires both a great measure of courage in the patient and an equal measure of confidence in one's physiotherapist. Bit by bit Jean coped well and increased her independent breathing to around four minutes – definitely a step in the right direction.

On about the tenth day while I was treating Jean, suddenly there was a great commotion. A young man was being rushed into the ward and both a porter and a nurse were hurrying to get an iron lung to bring over to the corner by the door. A doctor was with the patient when he called over to me to come quickly. I hurried across to the young man who was in a desperate condition, already blue in the face.

'Try and keep him breathing,' said the doctor handing me the portable respiratory apparatus, 'I'll have to give him another injection or we have lost him.'

I kept the young man ventilated as best I could while the doctor feverishly worked on him giving him another injection. The iron lung was opened and we all lifted the patient into it and he was sealed inside and the pump switched on. I turned away to go back to Jean when I suddenly remembered she was on a time trial breathing wise, and dashed over and switched on her pump. The look in her eyes as I returned to her told me all I needed to know. She had just managed to keep going, with certainly no breath left to call for help. I had been away for nearly five minutes.

'Jean!' I said horror struck at what had nearly happened. 'I am so very sorry about that.'

'It's alright now,' she said recovering as the pump worked its magic. 'I was desperately willing you to turn round to look at me and, thank goodness, you did and dashed over.' I stayed with her gently exercising her paralysed limbs, letting her talk her fright away. Jean had seen the whole emergency in her mirror and had heard the doctor call me over.

I felt quite shaken myself, at Jean's ordeal, yet the very nature of that unit meant that emergencies were a frequent happening during the height of the epidemic. Having lingered as long as I was able with Jean I said to her 'at least we know you can breathe for five minutes on your own!' I combed her hair before leaving and promising to be back during my lunch.

The young man, whom we had tried to keep alive, unfortunately did not last the hour. His poor wife was sitting in the hallway waiting to go in to him when I left. He was alive then but only just and she was nine months pregnant.

That was the nature of polio, sudden onset, gravity of the illness and all too frequent death. If the staff had not been so hectically busy, we might have been frightened for our own safety, as it was, it never crossed our minds.

My two weeks at the hospital rushed by and before I knew it was Friday afternoon. I went round saying goodbye to the patients, all of whom I knew by now. Some had made a good recovery and others were going on to their local hospital for intensive physio, to try to build up their residual muscle power and to be fitted with any supporting splints required. Lastly I went to the patients in the iron lungs and spent a few moments with each, they all wished me well in my coming finals and I in turn wished those brave people all the luck in the world, they would need it.

Ann had asked me what I intended to do once my exams were over saying that if I felt like it, she would be glad of my help until I had decided what I was going to do. I was delighted to be invited back, not least because Christmas would be coming up, and I promised I would return to help out as soon as I had finished my finals.

My last act at the hospital was to collect my pay packet of fourteen pounds from the office. That amounted to two weeks' pay, at the going rate of a newly qualified physiotherapist – I was wealthy.

CHAPTER FORTY

Fiona

I returned to Salford Royal on the following Monday morning, having promised Ann, at Monsall, I would return as soon as I had finished my exams. As I entered the hospital, I walked into Fiona, who greeted me and asked how had it gone? I told her about the work briefly as we walked along but I could see she was itching to tell me some news of her own.

'What?' I asked.

'I have met someone special' she whispered.

'Go on, tell me,' I asked, 'you must have ditched the horseman of wobbly Adam's apple and large feet fame?'

'Yes ages ago,' she continued. 'I was at a friend's wedding recently when I met Martin, he was one of the groomsmen. I was wearing a white fluffy hat with my outfit when he came up to me and said I looked like a newly hatched chick.' She laughed. 'He's quiet, a little shy, lives about twenty miles away and he is an accountant in his family's company,' Fiona said almost in one breath.

'What does the family company make?' I asked. 'It is bound to be something to do with cotton in that neck of the woods.'

'You are right,' Fiona said laughing. 'They make all sorts of surgical and hospital dressings, from now on I can get all the free ST's I need!'

'Handy,' I said laughing with my friend.

'No one here knows anything, I wanted you to be the first to know especially as I think we will be getting engaged soon. I have met his family, his mother is a bit formidable but really everyone is very nice and his family is catholic which helps.' I was certain that last bit of information, was the understatement of the year coming from Fiona and I was delighted 'things,' were going smoothly for her and said so. For a moment or two I felt a bit down, my great friend was about to get engaged, I felt like 'one green bottle left standing on the wall.' The moment soon passed though, there were more important things to think about right now.

Meanwhile, both the teaching and departmental staff were pulling out all the stops on our behalf. It was reassuring and gratifying to know everyone was doing the absolute utmost to ensure we would be successful. The department staff said they would let us know if they had anything of 'particular interest,' in their departments. Interesting, that in this context, meant any condition that was out of the ordinary or an unusual variation of a classical case, because the practical examinations were a vital part of the finals. They were a true indication of ones professional expertise, more so, perhaps, than the written papers.

'It is not that the straight forward classical cases were to be ignored that would have been downright fool hardy.' Bo had said in one of her final lectures. 'We all know some examiners like to test students, under pressure, and come up with some remote condition, just concentrate on the aims of the treatment, as far as that particular patient is concerned,' she advised. 'Amongst, the examiners there will be some who are specialists in their particular field, and they will undoubtedly ask questions about their speciality. Don't forget they probably have spent years researching and treating patients in their field of interest. What's more, with their extensive experience, they will be selective with their patients choosing those they know will respond to treatment. Stay calm, and try to remember patients that you most certainly will have treated with the same condition in your years here, and I know you will be all right. Good luck everyone,' said Bo spinning on her heel, as she left the final lecture – and that was that.

CHAPTER FORTY-ONE

Finals

The day dawned, cold and clear, with my chilblains giving me jip, and certainly not helping the little composure I had tried to build up.

Before leaving home, I checked I had my clean white coat and belt, scissors, pen, tape measure, hanky and hospital shoes. Many physiotherapy schools allowed their students to wear Clark's sandals but not Bo. For some reason, she insisted on brown lace up hospital shoes. In fact you could spot a 'foreign' physio a long way off by their footwear. Sadly, that particular style is not available anyway nowadays. We had finished our written finals - now for the practicals.

I arrived at the large teaching hospital, nervous yet anxious to get on with things. The hospital corridors were well marked with arrows and notices telling us which way to go.

We all met up in a large treatment area that had become our temporary changing room. The air was constrained as even friends hardly talked with one another. Fiona had been there some time because of her train timetable. Predictably she was sitting by herself quietly reading a pathology book.

'Hello,' I said glad to see her. 'Have you been here long?'

'Ten minutes,' she said, 'I was beginning to think I was the only one here, I'm frightened to death.'

'Well you certainly don't look it,' I replied, and she grinned.

'I have just seen Barbara, Sylvia and Paula, they have just popped down to the loo.' Fiona continued. 'By the way Sylvia is behaving, you would think she was totally incontinent.'

'Oh golly, I must go too before the rush,' I said, glad I wasn't the only one to be feeling that nervous.

I joined Fiona sitting down shaking out our starched white coats. It made all the difference. Putting on ones uniform you became instantly a physiotherapist and I for one, was certainly more in charge of my panic faculties. Our friends rejoined us and we all stood around waiting to be called.

Four students were called at any one time. Strict time keeping was in force anyone late was deemed to have failed outright. I heard my name and stepped forward with the three other candidates. A clipboard, carrying usher, opened the door of the examination hall and there we were, lambs to the slaughter.

The large room was quiet as we entered and in each corner there was a group of people stationed. Amongst the group was a student in gym kit, the nominal patient, and another presumably the reserve just in case, the examiner of course and a variety of apparatus. Along a sidewall sitting on a low gym bench, was a group of 'first years,' both men and women, along with some small apparatus presumably there in case an examiner wanted a demonstration of class taking.

All this I took in momentarily as the usher directed us to a particular corner. Standing in my particular corner, was a class or a group of students. I breathed a sigh of relief I was at home with class taking. My relief was short-lived. I was mistaken. I was not going to be asked to take a remedial class after all. The examiner asked me to take a student to a plinth. A strapping male student volunteered when he heard I needed a mid-thigh amputation.

'Now,' began the examiner, 'we have an elderly man here with circulatory problems. He has had a mid-thigh amputation, describe what you would expect to find first-day postoperative?' My mind went back to jolly Mr Sullivan, my patient some months ago at Hope hospital, a great comedian and therefore not easily forgotten. The thought of this cheery man collected my wits and I explained to the examiner that even before surgery I would have taught breathing exercises to prevent chest complications post-operatively and hip exercises to the hip extensors to prevent flexion of the stump.

'Show me,' said the examiner. I explained to my patient the need for breathing exercises to prevent him getting a post op chest infection, especially, I added, because you are a smoker. I went on to explain to the patient the need to do hip extension exercises prior to and post operatively, to prevent the stump, which would be minus weight of the lower leg after his operation, from flexing up. I went on to explain to my patient if he didn't do these exercises straight away post op., the powerful abductor and flexor muscles would work overtime forcing his stump up, making the fitting of an artificial limb and walking impossible.

The examiner continued to listen as I rattled on about correct bandaging to get the desired cone shape ready for the fitting of the prosthesis but made no comment. In desperation I went on to tell the patient about the possibility of experiencing pain in the amputated leg and that it was called phantom leg pain, due to parts of the nerve supply being still intact.

At last the examiner spoke and told me to move on to teaching my patient how to walk using his artificial limb, no easy task with an intact strapping male. The examiner watched and then asked me questions. Whilst he jotted down endless notes, my eyes rested on a student patient across the room, she was accurately portraying a 'stroke.' The exam candidate had clearly forgotten that a right handed stroke usually meant speech impairment but her young 'patient,' was helping her out as she gave an Oscar winning performance, by miming.

I was suddenly brought back to earth, by my examiner dismissing me with thanks, and directing me to another corner where a second examiner stood waiting for me. I thanked the man and walked away having no sense of how I had done at all. I was just suspended in time.

'Your patient is a young motor cyclist who was involved in a road traffic accident,' briskly stated the grey haired, pinched faced woman examiner in the second group. 'He had a badly trapped foot resulting in a torn Achilles tendon and serious ankle injuries, I want you to describe what torn structures might be involved around the 'sustem taculum tali.' As the examiner mentioned this particular bit of anatomy, she made it sound like an ancient incantation or perhaps something that is chanted whilst snaking round at a party, doing the rumba.

The wretched woman fixed me with her beady eye as I turned to the horror struck physio student, now motorcyclist. I pick up one of her feet taking it between both my hands pretending to examine the structures around the area, playing for thinking time. Like a bolt out of the blue, I heard myself describing it as I had chanted it rhythmically to myself in our kitchen at home, ages ago. I remembered it was that peculiar nob of bone on the instep. It was on the calcaneum, one of the large bones in the foot.

'Well,' said the angel of darkness, 'I am waiting.'

'Hmm,' I offered, 'there is likely to be injuries to the spring and deltoid ligaments and damage to the tendon of the flexor hallucis longus muscle.'

'Give me four alternative treatments,' she responded immediately. Oh lord, I am in the hands of a specialist I thought. I offered four possible treatments watching her eyes in the manner of a drowning man. Was it just possible that there was a flicker of enthusiasm when I mentioned ultrasound? Hoping I was on the right track I muttered something about megahertz and square pulses. The 'pinched' face looked questioningly at one suggestion so rather than expanding on that seemingly dangerous theme I quickly embarked on the additional merits of ice therapy. I was abruptly thanked and directed to the final corner.

I walked over to my next examiner who was a plump pleasant looking woman probably in her mid-forties. Her genial manner disguised her acute mind. Straight away she asked me some general questions about asthmatic children and how I'd teach relaxation. I began to explain and she cut me off, with a 'show me,' she said waving four athletic, very non-asthmatic students over. I asked the students to arrange themselves on the thin sponge mats on the floor, using a small pillow under their head. I then asked them to bend their knees so they would be relaxed, in the crook lying position. To warm up the class, I started out with deep gentle abdominal breathing with them sighing out as they exhaled.

I was just about to move on when the examiner abruptly stopped me and asked one of the female students to stand next to her, sending the others back to sit their bench by the wall. Wasting no time at all she said this woman had given birth to her third child four weeks previously. Although she was delighted to see her toes again for the first time in months, she had resulting poor posture, back ache and stress micturition. 'Tell me what are you going to do about it?' I saw the student look at me in a hapless sort of way. I was quite sure she didn't know the meaning of micturition, so there was no way that she could act the part. 'Micturition, means needing to spend a penny fast and frequently and is made embarrassingly worse in stressful conditions such as when coughing or sneezing,' I informed the student, at the same time letting my inquisitor know that I knew what we were talking about.

'The three conditions are all interlinked,' I said to the examiner. 'My patient needs posture exercises, which would include strengthening exercises to both the back and the abdomen with further specialised pelvic floor exercises to strengthen the peritoneal area.'

My mind went back to our early medical gym lectures with our gym lecturer, she of smokers cough and ankle twirling fame, who enthusiastically talked about bus stop exercises. These were simple, none obvious exercises that one had to do frequently to counter 'leakage' and could be done any time day and night, even whilst waiting for a bus she informed us. Basically they consisted of tightening one's abdominal muscles, clenching one's bottom and at the same time 'pulling up that area down below,' as our lecturer had delicately put it.

As my examiner looked on, I went through a selection of exercises that my patient would need to practise as often as she was able; bearing in mind she had three children to look after. But then that was the beauty of the bus stop exercise, I told my mother of three, that as well as at the bus stop, she could do the exercises standing at the cooker or at the kitchen sink, nobody will know.' As the examiner seemed interested in this I line of treatment, I advanced it as far as possible then added that 'of course I could offer a variety of electrical treatments such as ultra sound or diathermy, if the back ache persisted.' The examiner nodded and thanked me.

Was that it then, the final part of my exams? I walked to the door in a daze, completely drained. It was impossible to assess my performance, in any way. As I walked to the changing room, I was feeling vaguely depressed but most of all desperately tired. The changing room was empty except for two people whom I didn't know and judging from the empty pegs, several of my friends had left already. We had previously agreed to meet up some time later, so stepping out of my uniform and putting on my things I hurried out of the hospital.

CHAPTER FORTY-TWO

Monsall

I must have travelled home, but I didn't remember any of the journey or the fact it was pouring down with rain. I suddenly came to, standing at the front door searching in my handbag for my front door keys. My mother must have been watching out for me because before I could turn the key in the lock, she had opened the front door.

'Take your coat off and sit down,' my mother said looking at me, 'you look all in.' I did as I was told and returned to sit at the kitchen table where a piping hot cup of tea stood waiting for me. I was grateful to my mother for letting me sit and unwind, not asking me any questions just then. As my wise mother well knew, I would be glad to tell all, given time to recover. It was so lovely and comforting to sit there, being cosseted, so physically tired and mentally dazed, as I was.

'Don't think about work anymore,' my mother had said as she sat by me and laid her hands over mine. 'Just forget everything. We know you have done your best.'

I smiled my thanks at her reassuring words and as I finished my cup of tea she said,

'Go next door and have a rest it's lovely and warm.'

Next door, meant our drawing room, and as I entered, the warm cheery flicker of the fire was lighting up the room. I didn't switch on the light, there was no need, with the light of the open fire and the glow of the drawn, deep golden brown of the velvet curtains, closed against the faded light of the cold, wet October afternoon, it was everything a home should be. I settled back in the big, winged, leather armchair, with my feet curled up under me and fell fast asleep.

An hour later I heard the front door click shut and the drawing room door opened. My mother stood there, so like the Queen Mother in build and the way she would hold her head on the side.

'Feeling a bit better love?' She gently spoke.

'Much better thanks' I nodded and stretched, I had pins and needles in my feet because of the way I had fallen asleep.

'It had stopped raining,' my mother said, 'so I took Pandy out for a little walk to the park, the weather has been so bad we couldn't get out before.' Pandy who had been told to stay in the kitchen peeped round the door then seeing me, bolted in with his tail enthusiastically wagging in his endearing way. Yes I certainly felt better.

Later over our evening meal I told my family about the examinations and my mother chuckled over the bus stop exercises.

'Well that's that,' said my father, 'I'm sure everything will be fine but in any case it is pointless going over what might have been so forget it all and relax, you are taking the rest of the week off aren't you?'

'Yes,' I replied and for the rest of the week I sort of floated about in a dream like state helping my mother as needed but apart from that, as per instructions, I relaxed and felt much better for it.

The exam results were due out in two or three weeks so there would not be long to wait. I had spent the rest of the exam week doing nothing very much instead of all the lovely things I had promised myself, that I would do, somehow I just couldn't get my act together.

Roland came round, just to sit with me or to take me out which ever I preferred. He had listened to my account of my exams and had said nothing. He of course was a veteran of exams and knew only too well, what the tension was like but best of all he firmly, if silently, was convinced I would be successful.

The following Monday I returned to Monsall as promised. I had told Ann 'that I would help out until Christmas pass or fail,' the latter with Bo's permission. In any case Ann knew my stay would be temporary and that what I really wanted was a post in one of the large teaching hospitals, nearer my home in Manchester.

This arrangement suited everyone. With the colder weather, the epidemic was waning. By the end of October only very few new polio cases were being admitted. Those patients past the acute stage were being transferred to their local hospitals for on-going treatment, leaving only those patients who were still in their iron lungs.

Jean was one of those patients and I went to treat her on my first day back. Her breathing had continued to improve but it was clear she was gravely paralysed and would always remain so. Jean could manage independent breathing for up to ten minutes now she told me. It seemed so little but meant so much. She was hoping to go home soon for a trial run. Her husband was an able engineer, who already had plans and designs in force to help her live a little more independently. Eventually she left Monsall sometime after I did. Subsequently though, I did hear her husband had designed the first 'front loading' bath for the disabled as a consequence of his wife's disability and I just wished them all the luck in the world, they certainly deserved it.

I began to spend more time in the thoracic surgery wards, which in non emergency times, was where the main body of work was. This work was interspersed with my work on the ward for infants. Here very young children, mostly under two, had whooping cough. They too, by reason of age, were very ill. These babies in their large iron cots would be quite quiet one moment then one little mite would begin to cough, which soon developed into the typical prolonged whoop, as the baby fought for its breath. As soon as one child started it seemed to be the signal for all these tiny patients to cough and whoop ending with numerous exhausted babies crying and vomiting. Great care had to be taken to ensure the babies didn't inhale their vomit as they took in their long whooping gasps for air.

The days had past, more or less, routinely with no more polio patients being admitted. Polio seemed to have a preference for warmer weather, at any rate that is when the past epidemics seemed to have occurred. There was talk of a new vaccine from America, the Salk vaccine, taken by mouth, a few drops on a lump of sugar, totally painless and too late for the likes of Jean but what a gift to the world at large.

CHAPTER FORTY-THREE

Farewell Salford

Some three-weeks later, early in the morning my younger brother knocked on my bedroom door. John stood there in the doorway saying the post had just come. He was holding a thick brown envelope.

In a voice that was a mixture of apology and apprehension he hesitated to hand the envelope to me, the significance being that thick envelopes were supposed to contain a notice of failure and all the re-entry forms, but a thinner envelope contained only a letter of congratulations.

'Never mind,' I said to my anxious brother who was, by now, holding the envelope behind his back, 'give me the letter quickly.'

I opened the large buff envelope and took out several sheets of papers, at the same time thinking, I couldn't start all over again. I tried to focus my eyes. Yes I had passed. All the other papers were directions on paying annual subscriptions to The Chartered Society of Physiotherapy so I would not only have professional recognition but would also be insured to practise. There was another form to fill in, for confirmation I would be State registered, also at an annual fee. Clearly it was going to be expensive being not only being qualified, but actually staying qualified.

'It's alright,' I said to John who, still standing there and thinking the worst. 'I have passed!' A great smile of relieved pleasure swept across his face.

We rushed down to tell my parents the good news. They typically took the good news in their quiet, but clearly happy way, giving me a hug and a kiss, and a 'told you so.' I could hardly swallow my breakfast. I was anxious to get to Salford to meet my friends as previously agreed. Hopefully, we would all be congratulating ourselves and then collecting our personal things, or we would comfort and commiserate the unlucky.

I ran up the hospital steps, two at a time, glad to be meeting my friends but sad to be leaving the hospital. On the way to our common room, I met Bo and I was able to thank her in person for all the help she had given me, particularly in the last twelve months. She smiled and, after congratulating me, said that she too would be leaving soon.

'I am retiring,' she said, 'we are allowed to retire at fifty-five here and as I have been invited to start a new faculty of physiotherapy at Pretoria University in South Africa, that is where I am going.'

Now it was my time to offer her my congratulations and I wished her all the luck in the world in her new venture. We shook hands and wished each other all the best for the future.

I hurried on to the common room and saw everyone laughing and chatting. As Bo had mentioned in our brief conversation, everyone had been successful so there was great rejoicing all round. I told everyone of Bo's coming South African adventure, and we all heartily agreed she was indeed, someone very special.

Fiona whispered to me she and Martin were hoping to be married in spring next year and asked if I would be one of her bridesmaids. I gave her a hug and said I would be honoured to be included, and promised to meet up soon in any case.

I pushed open the heavy hospital doors of Salford Royal for the last time. I walked down the steps and turned left, onto busy Chapel Street. I passed the few shops that remained on this main arterial road, most of which were either pawn shops or those selling cheap clothing some, second, even third hand.

As I walked along the busy road, I couldn't help think of my awful, disjointed start. I had not wanted to return. For me, it certainly had been a resisted exercise, but as I had learnt, resisted exercises are strengthening exercises. I did feel strong, I felt independent but most importantly of all, I felt happy and content.

I passed the derelict alehouse belonging to yesteryear and crossed the road at the traffic lights and headed down to Bridge Street. I worked my way through the small side streets along the route that I had perfected in the last three years, walking from the city of Salford into the city of Manchester, to Piccadilly.

Jumping on my waiting bus, I sat down by a window and settling back stared out of the bus window. I saw nothing. I just looked forward, with pleasurable anticipation, to my future.